12 KEYS TO A HEALTHIER CANCER PATIENT

Unlocking your body's
incredible ability to heal itself
while working with your doctor

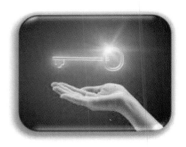

Patrick Quillin

Nutrition Times Press, Inc.

Copyright 2019

ISBN 978-0-578-56429-6

Printed in the United States of America.

Bulk purchases of this book available through:
Bookmasters, 800-247-6553

Nutrition Times Press, Inc.
Box 130789
Carlsbad, CA 92013
Ph.760-804-5703
Email: support@gettinghealthier.com

Table of Contents

Dedicated to

My mother,
Margaret Mary Quillin (b.1927-).
For bringing me into this world,
and raising me with respect,
and reading to me when younger,
and sharing your passion for the Divinely
orchestrated beauty and wisdom found in
nature.

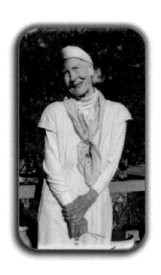

Thank You!

Camille Hughes, for your awesome computer talents in making
this book a professional package.

R. Michael Williams, MD, PhD, for inviting me into this
challenging and rewarding work of helping cancer patients.

Dick Stephenson and Bob Mayo, for your tutelage and support
in my 10 years at Cancer Treatment Centers of America.

Alan Gaby, MD and Jonathan Wright, MD, for your courage
and intellect in bringing credibility to nutritional medicine.

Ty and Charlene Bollinger,
for your brilliant and
relentless quest to bring The
Truth About Cancer to the
public.

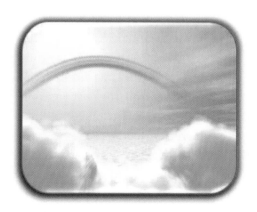

Preface

We live in a golden age of inventions and discoveries. Your smartphone has more computing power than the mainframe computers at the Social Security Administration in the 1950s. Moore's law speaks of the doubling of computing power every two years. Satellite communications, GPS for 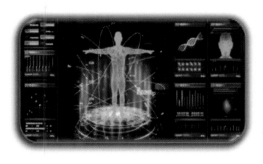 directions, the staggering capabilities of the internet are examples of our modern technological accomplishments. Medicine has been keeping pace with technology. Telemedicine has a specialist thousands of miles away reading radiology results for the patient. 3D printing allows doctors to make custom spare parts for a human. Robotic surgery takes away the limitations of imperfect human surgery. Lasik, hip and knee replacements, dialysis, deciphering the DNA, targeted drugs. Pain management drugs to allow millions to live in relative comfort. All well and good.

The dark side of technology is that we developed the naïve assumption that modern humans have transcended the laws of nature. That we can live on cadaver foods full of chemicals with no nourishment. That we can stare at a screen for 10 hours a day and not suffer the consequences. That we can live in a polluted and stress filled environment and not reap the harvest from our lifestyle.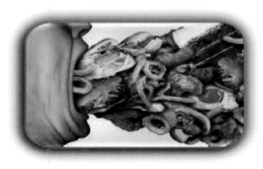

88% of Americans have some metabolic disorder. 2/3 of Americans are overweight. The incidence of diabetes has skyrocketed from the rare rich obese man to now 30 million Americans have it and another 60 million are prediabetic. Nearly 6 million Americans have Alzheimer's

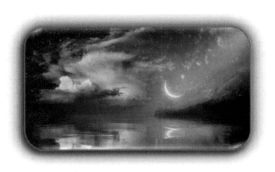

disease. In one generation autism incidence has grown from 1 in 5000 to now 1 in 59. Cancer incidence has increased from 1% of deaths in 1900 to 24% of deaths in 2017. Technology and our modern lifestyle have come with a cost.

In spite of the extraordinary developments of our modern culture, we are still a billion-year old carbon. The needs and limitations of our body has not changed measurably since the first human emerged 2 million years ago. We ignore our ingrained biological needs and

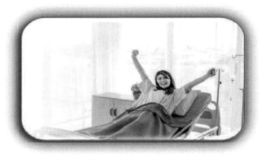

pump $480 billion worth of toxic prescription medications into our bodies in a futile attempt to subdue symptoms resulting from ignoring the laws of nature. But fear not. There are answers to many of the above health dilemmas and they are evidence-based, simple, cheap, and easy to incorporate into your lifestyle.

This book is about your healing from cancer while working with your doctor. Everything mentioned in this book is meant to buttress your doctor's best care, not to replace it. Let's be clear. I do not cure anyone. I am an educator with a rare grasp of the keys required to unlock your body's unfathomable healing capacity. Your true doctor lives within you. And together, we are going to bring your innate healing capacity up to its peak.

This book was 14 years in the making. This book is meant to be an advanced companion to my 2005 bestseller, BEATING CANCER WITH NUTRITION. This book is a consolidation of my 20 years of education, 40 years of professional experience, thousands of patients that I counselled, hundreds of textbooks that I have read, thousands of peer reviewed journal articles I have read, and over 600 hours of postgraduate training at seminars. Do not underestimate the power in this information.

The feedback I received over the past years has helped to shape this book into its format. Plenty of color illustrations are used. "A picture is worth a thousand words." And a lot easier and more enjoyable to grasp. Large type is used since many cancer patients are older and may have compromised vision. No words are wasted in this book. Words are simply tools to bridge the gap between my mind and your mind. I am not trying to impress anyone with my vocabulary, but simply choosing the proper tool for the job.

Each of these chapters could have been a semester class in college rich in bombastic scientific language. I have spared you the trouble. This book is interactive. Those who are reading the e-book or Kindle version will be able to click on hyperlinks to visit the original 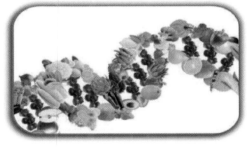 study or website. This book is meant to provide you with a short, punchy, easy to read, colorful, bullet point guide to get your body back into prime healing mode. Without further ado, let's do this.

KEY 1
UNDERSTAND THE PROBLEM

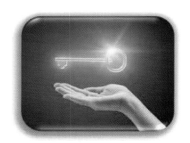

Chapter 1
War on Cancer: a Qualified Failure

"Modern medicine is based on a lie."
Dale Bredesen, MD, author of bestselling book THE END OF ALZHEIMER'S

<u>*FROM NATURE'S PHARMACY: Phytic Acid*</u>

IP6 and protease inhibitors. Did nature make a mistake? Whole grains and legumes contain a substance called phytic acid, which binds up minerals, especially iron, and escorts them out of the system. Phytic acid is a seed's way of storing phosphorus, like a school lunch bucket. For decades in the later 20th century, nutritionists thought that phytic acid must have been some mistake or "anti-nutrient" in whole grains and legumes, hence providing even more enthusiasm for processing grains down to white flour. In fact, we now find that phytic acid is one of the key ingredients in plant food lowering the risk for <u>various cancers, kidney stones, heart disease, and liver disease</u>.[1] Best sources include beans, brown rice, sesame seeds, and corn. Phytic acid is now sold as a nutrition supplement: IP6, inositol hexaphosphate 6. In a similar vein, protease inhibitors are substances in legumes, especially soybeans, which can inhibit enzymes that break down protein in the gut. Again, nutritionists thought of protease inhibitors as "anti-nutrients". Raw legumes are unhealthy. However, there is now compelling evidence that these protease inhibitors actually are very therapeutic in retarding cancer growth, and even allowing humans to better

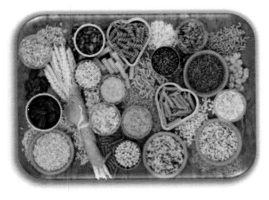

tolerate radiation without serious side effects. Protease inhibitor drugs are now the fashionable trend in the pharmaceutical industry in slowing down the growth of viruses, including AIDS. Nature knows what it is doing. Do not bet against the wisdom of whole foods.

This chapter is intended to provide a wakeup call for cancer patients. While your oncologist is likely to recommend chemo, radiation, and/or surgery; there is compelling evidence that these therapies are not enough to give you the best chance of remission or even extension of lifespan. This chapter is your roadmap to augment your doctor's best care in providing integrative health care while undergoing conventional cancer treatment.

Cancer is not a new phenomenon. Archeologists have discovered tumors on dinosaur skeletons and Egyptian mummies. From 1600 B.C. on, historians find records of attempts to treat cancer. In the naturalist Disney film, "Never Cry Wolf", the biologist sent to the Arctic to observe the behavior of wolves found that the wolves would kill off the easiest prey, which were sometimes animals suffering from leukemia. Cancer is an abnormal and rapidly growing tissue, which, if unchecked, will eventually smother the body's normal processes. Cancer may have been with us from the beginning of time, but the fervor with which it attacks modern civilization is unprecedented. There will be 1.7 million new cases of cancer in 2018 with 609,000 deaths.

Magic Bullets vs. Real Healing

When Richard Nixon launched the "war on cancer" in 1971, he claimed that we would have a cure for a major cancer by the Bicentennial of 1976. That cure was to be accomplished just like the space race, in which America threw its prodigious funding and genius behind putting a man on the moon by 1969. That was accomplished.

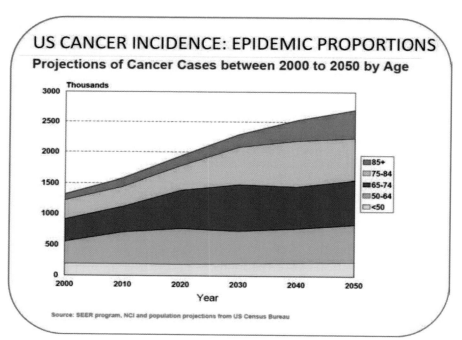

The war on cancer has been, at best, a qualified failure, and at worst, an unmitigated disaster. The difference between the war on cancer and the space race was errors in thinking. The space race created solid state transistors, computers, and many other incredibly valuable technological breakthroughs in order to accomplish their task. The war on cancer stood on the thin ice of finding a magic bullet against cancer, just like antibiotics seemed to cure certain bacterial infections. There is a huge difference between the occasional dazzling cure for a bacterial infection vs. trying to find a magic bullet drug that would cure cancer. Cancer is an abnormal growth that exists in the patient due to abnormal conditions.

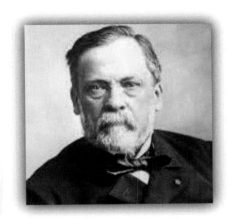

Louis Pasteur, French biologist and one of the first scientific "rock stars" of the modern era spent his life trying to eradicate, or Pasteurize, as many microbes as possible. In the end, Pasteur conceded "I have been wrong. The germ is nothing. The "terrain" is everything." The terrain is where the germ or cancer starts. Changing the underlying causes of cancer is both complex and crucial for long term success in curing cancer. Modern oncology ignores this obvious fact.

Richard Nixon declared "war on cancer" on December 23, 1971. Nixon confidently proclaimed that we would have a cure for cancer within 5 years, by the 1976 Bicentennial. However, by 1991, a group of 60 noted physicians and scientists gathered a press conference to tell the public "The cancer establishment confuses the public with repeated claims that we are winning the war on cancer... Our ability to treat and cure most cancers has not materially improved."[2] The unsettling bad news is irrefutable:

⇒ newly-diagnosed cancer incidence continues to escalate, from 1.1 million Americans in 1991 to 1.6 million in 2017

⇒ deaths from cancer in 2018 were 613,000, up from 514,000 in 1991

⇒ since 1950, the overall cancer incidence has increased by 44%, with breast cancer and male colon cancer up by 60% and prostate cancer by 100%

⇒ for decades, the 5 year survival has remained constant, for non-localized breast cancer at 18% and lung cancer at 13%

⇒ only 5% of the $5.7 billion annual budget for the National Cancer Institute is spent on prevention

⇒ grouped together, the average cancer patient has a 50/50 chance of living another 5 years, which are the same odds he or she had in 1971

⇒ claims for cancer drugs are generally based on tumor response rather than prolongation of life. Many tumors will initially shrink when chemo and radiation are applied, yet tumors often develop drug-resistance and are then unaffected by therapy.

⇒ within the next few years, cancer is expected to eclipse heart disease as the number one cause of death in America. It is already the number one fear. 42% of Americans living today can expect to develop cancer

Have We Made Any Progress?

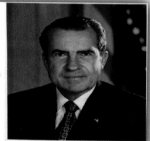

Key 1:
Recognize the problem
Failures in the
"war on cancer"
"We will have a cure for a major cancer by the bi-centennial celebration of the United States."
Richard Nixon 1971
48 years later and over $200 billion in research
$4 trillion in treatment. Still no cures for cancer

Time for Examining Options

PROGRESS REPORT IN THE WAR ON CANCER

Chemotherapy is curative in about 2% of advanced
cancer. Guy Faguet, MD, 2005 WAR ON CANCER
ANATOMY OF FAILURE

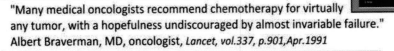

"Many medical oncologists recommend chemotherapy for virtually
any tumor, with a hopefulness undiscouraged by almost invariable failure."
Albert Braverman, MD, oncologist, *Lancet, vol.337, p.901, Apr.1991*

Chemotherapy is unsatisfactory; responses are rarely complete,
five year survival rates [for metastatic melanoma] are less than 5%,
and chemotherapeutic agents are toxic and expensive."
Morton, DL, et al, CA Cancer Journal Clinicians (ACS), vol.49, p.101, Mar.1999

"Chemotherapy is effective in about 3% of advanced epithelial cancers.
A sober analysis of the literature has rarely revealed any therapeutic success
by the chemotherapeutic regimens in question." *Abel, Hippocrates Verlag, 1990*

IN SPITE OF THIS DATA, CHEMO, RAD TX, & SURGERY
ARE ONLY ACCEPTED REIMBURSABLE CANCER TX IN US
"Nutrition reduces the effectiveness of chemo & rad tx???."

The purpose of this section is not to blast the National Cancer Institute, but rather to make it blatantly obvious that our current cancer treatment methods are inadequate and incomplete and that we need to examine some options--like nutrition. Also, we need to address the urgent question: "Does nutrition reduce the effectiveness of chemotherapy?" There are two parts to this debate.

1) Does nutrition interfere with chemotherapy? "No."
2) Is chemotherapy effective? The answer is "sometimes".

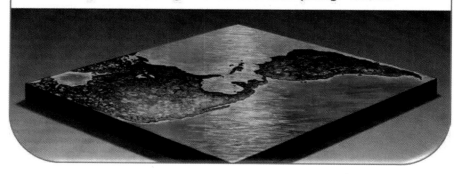

PARADIGM SHIFTS TAKE TIME
the world is flat
what you can't see can't hurt you
USDA food pyramid + RDA nutrition = good health
cancer is irreversible; therapies must be highly toxic
"The germ is nothing. The terrain is everything." Pasteur

Is Chemo Effective?

When examining risk to benefit to cost ratio of chemo for cancer patients, we find that the side effects for most chemo drugs as listed on the Mayo Clinic website include: damage to heart, lungs, kidneys, nerves (causing painful neuropathy), inducing cancer, and the routine nausea, vomiting, hair loss, fever, loss of appetite, bruising, immune suppression, and more. So the risks are high. What are the benefits? There have been many studies showing the relative ineffectiveness of chemo in treating cancer. One of the more respected published articles showed that chemo works in about 2% of all cancer patients.[3] Yet chemo is given to nearly 2/3 of cancer patients. And chemo may even cause the cancer to spread or metastasize.[4]

As a percentage of total annual deaths in America, cancer has escalated from 3% in 1900 to 24% of today's deaths. Many experts have been quick to explain away this frightening trend by claiming that our aging population is responsible for the increase in cancer incidence--older people are more likely to get cancer. But aging does not entirely explain our epidemic proportions of cancer in America.

Not that money should be a top priority when health and life are at stake, but our health costs are out of control. We spend about $3.5 trillion per year or 17% of our gross national product on health care, compared to Sweden at 8%, a socialistic country with free health care for all, and compared to our former American level of 3% in the year 1900. Even after adjusting for inflation, we spend twice as much money on health care for the elderly as we did prior to the inauguration of Medicare.[5] Cancer care is the most expensive of all diseases, costing Americans about $150 billion annually, not including lost work time etc.

SHIFTING THE CANCER PARADIGM
MUST WE KILL TO CURE?
Journal of Clinical Oncology (ASCO), vol.13, no.4, p.801, Apr.1995
H. Schipper, CR Goh, TL Wang

"the limits of the [cancer killing] model seem to have been reached"

"consider cancer as potentially reversible"

"killing strategies may be counterproductive because they impair host response and drive the already defective regulatory process [of the cancer cell] toward further aberrancy."

"[chemotherapy] treatment strategies have been based on the log-cell kill hypothesis, derived from leukemia cells in culture...but is rarely seen in nature and only sustained under stringent conditions"

"remission does not predict cure...the failure of adjuvant therapies to flatten disease-free survival curves"

"conventional antineoplastic approaches will play a role as debulkers, ...the strategy will change to one of reregulation."

Ulrich Abel, PhD, of the Heidelberg Tumor Center in Germany, has brought the issue to a fever pitch. Abel, a well-respected biostatistics expert, published a controversial 92-page review of the world's literature on survival of chemotherapy-treated cancer patients, showing that chemotherapy alone can help only about 3% of the patients with epithelial cancer (such as breast, lung, colon, and prostate), which kills 80% of total cancer patients. "...a sober and unprejudiced analysis of the literature has rarely revealed any therapeutic success by the regimens in question."[6]

Breast and prostate cancers have recently surfaced in the press as "forgotten cancers", due to their intimate nature. While one out of 20 women in 1950 were hit with breast cancer, today that number is one in eight. Even with early detection and proper treatment, a "cured" breast cancer patient will lose an average of 19 years of lifespan. Breast cancer kills about 45,000 women each year.[7] Lack of faith in cancer treatment has led a few physicians to recommend that some women with a high incidence of breast or ovarian cancer in their family undergo "preventive surgery" to remove these high-risk body parts.[8] Life and health insurance companies now refer to healthy intact women as "with organs" and at high risk, therefore forced to pay higher health insurance premiums.

COMMON MISCONCEPTIONS AMONG ONCOLOGISTS

MYTH: Nutrition has nothing to do with cancer.

FACT: The health of all animals and plants is heavily dependent on nutrition. Nutrition improves outcome in cancer treatment.

MYTH: Antioxidants are both expensive urine and will neutralize the benefits of chemo and radiation.

FACT: Then why are the antioxidant drugs Amifostine (cisplatin), Mesna (Ifosphomide), and Dextrazazone (Adria) used with chemo?

MYTH: Sugar has nothing to do with cancer outcome.

FACT: Then why is the $1.5 million PET scan considered such a valuable tool in diagnosing cancer?

While Tamoxifen is an estrogen binder that can be of benefit in short-term use for breast cancer patients and it has been touted as a chemo-preventive agent for millions of high-risk breast cancer patients, other data show that long-term tamoxifen use elevates the risk for heart attack,[9] eye,[10] and liver damage[11] and INCREASES the risk of endometrial cancer.[12]

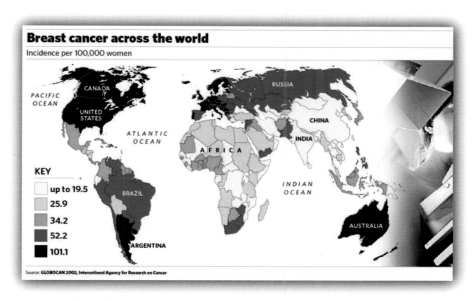

Breast cancer across the world
Incidence per 100,000 women

KEY
up to 19.5
25.9
34.2
52.2
101.1

Source: GLOBOCAN 2002, International Agency for Research on Cancer

And while breast cancer is tragic, prostate cancer is equally prevalent in men and even more lethal. The NCI spends one fourth the amount on prostate cancer research as on breast cancer research. The prostate specific antigen (PSA) and digital rectal exam are the early screening procedures for prostate cancer. In the majority of prostate cancers found, the cancer has spread beyond the prostate gland and is difficult to treat. Comparing the outcome of 223 patients with untreated prostate cancer to 58 patients who underwent radical prostatectomy, the 10-year disease-specific survival was 86.8% and 87.9%, respectively. There was essentially no difference in survival between the treated and untreated groups.[13]

According to an extensive review of the literature, there has been no improvement in cancer mortality from 1952 through 1985.[14] These authors state: "Evidence has steadily accrued that [cancer therapy] is essentially a failure." Meanwhile, we spend millions researching molecular biology in a futile quest for a "magic bullet" against cancer.[15] A London physician and researcher has provided statistical backing for his contention that breast cancer screenings in women under age 50 provide no benefit in 99.85% of the premenopausal women tested.[16] The average cancer patient has only a 60% chance of surviving the next five years— slightly better than survival rates from 30 years ago. A gathering chorus of scientists and clinicians proclaim that success from chemo and radiation therapy has plateaued, and that we need to examine alternative therapies.[17]

A 1971 textbook jointly published by the American Cancer Society and the University of Rochester stated that biopsy of cancer tissue may lead to the spread of cancer.[18] Although encapsulated cancer can be effectively treated with surgery, and 22% of all cancer can be "cured" through surgery[19], 30% or more of surgery patients with favorable prognosis still have cancer recurrences.[20] A study of 440,000 cancer patients who received chemotherapy or radiation showed that those treated with radiation had a significantly increased risk for a type of leukemia involving cells other than the lymphocytes.[21] Long-term effects of radiation include birth defects and infertility. Short-term effects include mouth sores and ulcers, which can interfere with the ability to eat, rectal ulcers, fistulas, bladder ulcers, diarrhea, and colitis.

In a survey of 79 Canadian oncologists, all of them would encourage patients with non-small cell lung cancer to participate in a chemotherapy protocol, yet 58% said that they themselves would not participate in such a therapy and 81% said they would not take cisplatin (a chemo drug) under any circumstances.[22]

Analysis of over 100 clinical trials using chemotherapy as sole treatment in breast cancer patients found no benefits and significant damage from the chemotherapy in post-menopausal patients.[23] Dr. Rose Kushner pointed out that toxic drugs are "literally making healthy people sick" and are "only of marginal benefit to the vast majority of women who develop breast cancer."[24] Some evidence indicates that chemotherapy actually shortens the life of breast cancer patients.[25] New evidence shows that chemo not only does not help, but may spread breast cancer through metastasis.[26]

According to a psychologist writing in the American Cancer Society Journal, "the side effects of cancer chemotherapy can cause more anxiety and distress than the disease itself."[27] A well-recognized side effect of chemotherapy is suppression of bone marrow, which produces the white blood cells that fight infection. This common immune suppression leads to the all-too-common death from infection.[28]

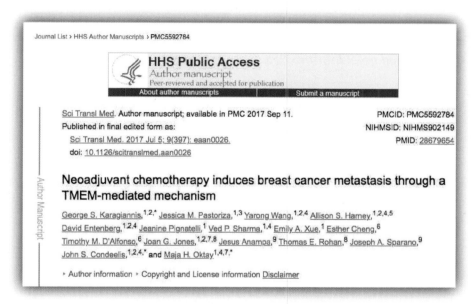

According to the literature that comes with each chemotherapeutic agent, methotrexate may be "hepatotoxic" (damaging to the liver) and suppresses immune function. Adriamycin can cause "serious irreversible myocardial toxicity (damage to heart) with delayed congestive heart failure often unresponsive to any cardiac supportive therapy." Cytoxan can cause "secondary malignancies" (cancer from its use). It is widely known among health care professionals that just working around chemotherapy agents can cause birth defects.[29]

In spite of $200 billion in research at the NCI and billions more spent in private industry, there have been few new chemotherapy drugs discovered in the past 20 years.[30] Not even NCI official Dr. Daniel Ihde can conjure up any enthusiasm for the failure of chemotherapy drugs against lung cancer.[31] Given the limited successes in traditional cancer treatment, it is not surprising that over 60% of all American cancer patients seek "alternative therapies".

Biological therapies, such as interferon and interleukin, are extremely toxic, with treatment requiring weeks of hospitalization, usually in intensive therapy, with multiple transfusions, severe bleeding, shock, and confusion as common side effects.[32] Interferon causes rapid onset of fever, chills, and severe muscle contractions that may require morphine.[33]

Financial Meltdown of Modern Medicine
"No good deed goes unpunished." Anonymous

In the dark days of World War II, America was struggling to climb out of the decade of financial depression while fighting a war on two continents. Most able-bodied young men went to war. Women, like my grandmother, worked in the factories to provide supplies to the war movement. In order to prevent inflation, the federal government mandated wage freezes. Yet manufacturers had contracts with the government to produce airplanes, ships, and all the other needs of war. Employers started offering "free health care" as an incentive to bring capable workers to their factories. Seemed like an innocent idea at the time, but it has become a Frankenstein in America that threatens to bring the world's greatest government to its knees. Once the war was over, the concept of free health care as a "perk" (perquisite) grew in popularity, especially among union jobs. Once Mom and Dad had free healthcare, the next step was getting free health care for Grandma and Grandpa, which began with the passage of the Medicare Act in 1965. We need to take care of our senior citizens. Yet America has lost the concept of "personal accountability" that founded this country and put us at the top of the world's caste system. Health care in general and cancer treatment in specific threaten our way of life unless we can get a handle on more cost effective and humane ways to treat cancer.

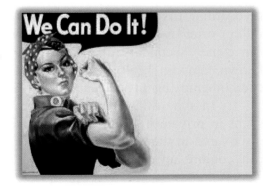

Social Security becomes an "unsecured liability" in the very near future, meaning "we have no clue where the money will come from to support it". Medicare is even more immediately perched on the brink of financial ruin. We currently spend a billion dollars a day on Medicare, of which 60% goes to treat patients in their last 6 months of life, with questionable results in either quality or quantity of life. Our $3.5 trillion per year health care system equates to $10,700 per person or 18% of gross domestic product…an unsustainable number by everyone's verdict. These unrealistic health care costs are added on to the cost of producing goods and services in America and has made America far less competitive in the global economy, costing us millions of jobs, which are "outsourced"

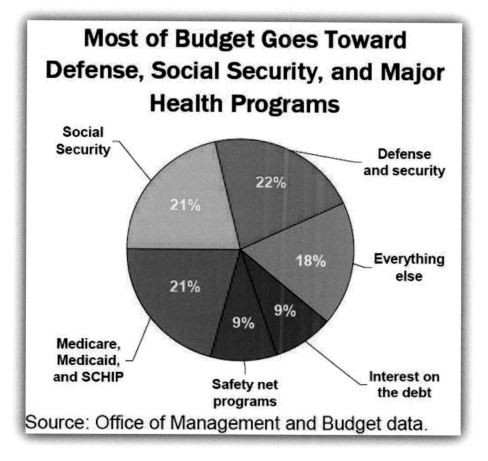

overseas. General Motors spends more on health care insurance for its employees than on the steel going into your car.

As you can see from the accompanying graphs found at the Government Accountability Office (GAO.gov), Social Security and Medicare are already the largest expenses in the federal budget and, with the aging of the 75 million baby boomers, threaten the solvency of the American government. We need more effective and more economical ways of dealing with disease. Nutrition tops that list.

Where Did We Go Wrong?

There is a lot of finger-pointing since the war on cancer has been so heavily criticized. For starters, it would be easy to blame bread mold, from which springs penicillin, which was discovered by Alexander Fleming in 1928 and gave us hope that there was a "magic bullet" against every disease. We could rest equal blame on Jonas Salk, inventor of the polio vaccine in 1952, for such a tremendous show from his medicine bag. With a simple vaccine, one of the most tragic pandemic plagues of history was felled. Again, more reasons to believe that a "magic bullet" against every disease must exist.

Another scapegoat is good old patriotic pride. After all, it was the Americans who rode in to World Wars I and II to rescue the world. Americans stepped in to finish the Panama Canal after the French had failed. Americans threw enough money at the Manhattan Project to develop a war-ending nuclear bomb and again bought our way to the moon in a massive and expensive effort from NASA scientists. Americans have more patents and Nobel laureates than any other nation on earth. We had good reasons to be confident of buying a cure for cancer.

Some of our problems lie in scientific research models. Using animals with induced leukemia, a non-localized disease of the blood-forming organs, is not a realistic representation of how well a cancer drug will work against a solid human tumor. We have also made the erroneous assumption that "no detectable cancer" means no cancer. A million cancer cells are undetectable by even the most sensitive medical equipment. A billion cancer cells become a tiny and nearly undetectable "lump".[34] When the surgeon says, "We think we got it all."--that is when the war on cancer must become an invisible battle involving the patient's well-nourished immune system.

We also have wrongly guessed that "response rate", or shrinkage of the tumor, is synonymous with cure. As mentioned, chemotherapy works on cancer cells like pesticides work on insects. Spraying pesticides on a field of plants may kill 99% of the bugs in the field, but the few insects that survive this baptism of poison have a unique genetic advantage to resist the toxicity of the pesticide. These "super bugs" then reproduce even more rapidly without competition, since the pesticides killed off biological predators in the field and reduced the fertility of the soil for an overall drop in plant health. Similarly, blasting a typically malnourished cancer patient with bolus (high dose once per week) injections of chemotherapy alone may elicit an initial shrinkage of the tumor, but the few tumor cells that survive this poison become resistant to therapy and may even accelerate the course of the disease in the now immune-suppressed patient. Meanwhile, the once marginally malnourished patient becomes clinically malnourished, since nausea becomes a prominent symptom in bolus chemo usage. An expert in cancer at Duke University, Dr. John Grant, has estimated that 40% or more of cancer patients actually die from malnutrition.[35]

We also made the mistake of becoming enamored with a few tools that we thought could eradicate cancer. We focused all of our energies in these three areas and ridiculed or even outlawed any new ideas. The real reason for our failure lies in our error in thinking. The wellness and illness of our bodies are almost entirely dependent on what we eat, think, drink, breathe, and how we move. These forces shape our general metabolism, which is the sum total of bodily processes. Our metabolism then either favors or discourages the growth of both infectious and degenerative diseases. Cancer is a degenerative disease of abnormal metabolism throughout the body--not just a regionalized lump or bump.

Our health is composed of a delicate interplay of nutrients consumed and toxins expelled, coupled with mental and spiritual forces that influence metabolism. We are a product of our genes, lifestyle, and environment. We are not dumb automobiles to be taken to the mechanic and fixed. We are physical and metaphysical beings who must become part of the cure, just as surely as we are a part of the disease process.

Healing is a joint effort between patient, clinician, and that mysterious and wonderful force which most of us take for granted. The days of "magic bullet" cures are over. The days of cooperative efforts between patient and clinician are here to stay.

Only Teamwork Will Beat Cancer

Cancer is now the number one or two cause of death in America. Cancer is a cruel disease that infiltrates the body with abnormal tissue growth and finally strangles its victims with malnutrition, infections, or multiple organ failure.

We need teamwork in cancer treatment because of the formidable "Predator" that we face. We cannot discard any cancer therapy, no matter how strange or perpendicular to medical theories, unless that therapy does not work. There are no "magic bullets" against cancer, nor can we anticipate such a development within our lifetime. We need to use restrained chemo, radiation, hyperthermia, and surgery to debulk the tumors, which can remove 10 or 20 trillion cancer cells and give the cancer patient's system a fighting 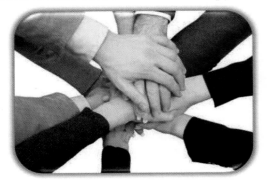 chance. At the same time, we need to re-regulate the cancer back toward healthy cooperation in the body with agents like protease enzymes.[36] Then we need to apply nutrition and other naturopathic fields to bolster "non-specific host defense mechanisms" in the cancer patient to reverse the underlying cause of the disease. This threefold approach, reduction of tumor burden without harming the patient, re-regulating the cancer to convert to normal healthy tissue, and nourishing the patient's recuperative powers, will be the humane and clinically effective cancer treatment of the new millennium.

Chemotherapy can be useful, especially for certain types of cancer and when administered in fractionated dose or via intra-arterial infusion to a therapeutically-nourished patient. Radiation therapy has its place, especially as the highly-targeted brachytherapy or intensity modulated radiation therapy (IMRT). Surgery has its place, especially when the tumor has been encapsulated and can be removed without bursting the collagen envelope. Hyperthermia can be extremely valuable. Combinations of these traditional therapies are becoming better accepted in medical circles. Later in this book, you will see the synergism in creative combinations of conventional and unconventional cancer therapies, *such* as quercetin (a bioflavonoid) with heat therapy, or niacin with radiation therapy. The take-home lesson here is: "Just because traditional medicine has failed to develop an unconditional cure for cancer doesn't mean that we should categorically reject all traditional approaches."

Comprehensive cancer treatment uses traditional cancer therapies to reduce the tumor burden, while concurrently building up the "terrain" of the cancer patient to fight the cancer on a microscopic level. That is the "one-two punch" that will eventually bring the predator of cancer to its knees.

PATIENT PROFILE:

L.M. was diagnosed in 1994 with late stage breast cancer. She read and followed the principles in BEATING CANCER WITH NUTRITION while using her doctor's selective tumor debulking therapies. While her prognosis had been poor, L.M. went into complete remission. L.M. attended a lecture by your author in Atlanta in November of 2018 and was delighted with her newfound health. 25 years after her death sentence, L.M. looks and feels fabulous.

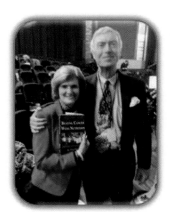

ENDNOTES

[1] https://www.ncbi.nlm.nih.gov/pubmed/22993910
[2] Ingram, B., Medical Tribune, vol.33, no.4, p.1, Feb.1992
[3] https://www.ncbi.nlm.nih.gov/pubmed/15630849
[4] https://stm.sciencemag.org/content/9/397/eaan0026
[5] Stout, H, Wall Street Journal, p.B5, Feb.26, 1992
[6] Abel, U., CHEMOTHERAPY OF ADVANCED EPITHELIAL CANCER: A Critical Survey, Hippokrates Verlag Stuttgart, 1990
[7] Neuman, E, New York Times, Insight, p.7, Feb.9, 1992
[8] Bartimus, T., Tulsa World, p.B3, Dec.22, 1991
[9] Nakagawa, T., et al., Angiology, vol.45, p.333, May 1994
[10] Pavlidis, NA, et al., Cancer, vol.69, p.2961, 1992
[11] Catherino, WH, et al., Drug Safety, vol.8, p.381, 1993
[12] Seoud, MAF, et al., Obstetrics & Gynecology, vol.82, p.165, Aug.1993
[13] Johansson, JE, et al., Journal American Medical Association, vol.267, p.2191, Apr.22, 1992
[14] Temple, NJ, et al., Journal Royal Society Medicine, vol.84, p.95, 1991
[15] Temple, NJ, et al., Journal Royal Society of Medicine, vol.84, p.95, Feb.1991
[16] Shaffer, M., Medical Tribune, p.4, Mar.26, 1992
[17] Hollander, S., et al., Journal of Medicine, vol.21, p.143, 1990
[18] Rubin, P., (ed), CLINICAL ONCOLOGY FOR MEDICAL STUDENTS AND PHYSICIANS: A MULTI-DISCIPLINARY APPROACH, 3rd edition, Univ. Rochester, 1971
[19] American Cancer Society, "Modern cancer treatment" in CANCER BOOK, Doubleday, NY, 1986
[20] National Cancer Institute, Update: Primary treatment is not enough for early stage breast cancer, Office of Cancer Communications, May 18, 1988
[21] Curtis, RE, et al., Journal National Cancer Institute, p.72, Mar.1984
[22] Ginsberg, RJ, et al., Cancer of the lung, in: DeVita, CANCER PRINCIPLES AND PRACTICES OF ONCOLOGY, Lippincott, Philadelphia, p.673, 1993

[23] New England Journal Medicine, Feb.18, 1988; see also Boffey, PM, New York Times, Sept.13, 1985

[24] Kushner, R., CA-Cancer Journal for Clinicians, p.34, Nov.1984

[25] Powles, TJ, et al., Lancet, p.580, Mar.15, 1980

[26] https://www.ncbi.nlm.nih.gov/pmc/articles/PMC5592784/

[27] Redd, WH, CA-Cancer Journal for Clinicians, p.138, May1988

[28] Whitley, RJ, et al., Pediatric Annals, vol.12, p.6, June 1983; see also Cancer Book, ibid.

[29] Jones, RB, et al., California Journal of American Cancer Society, vol.33, no.5, p.262, 1983

[30] Hollander, S., and Gordon, M., Journal of Medicine, vol.21, no.3, p.143, 1990

[31] Ihde, DC, Annals of Internal Medicine, vol.115, no.9, p.737, Nov.1991

[32] Moertel, CG, Journal American Medical Association, vol.256, p.3141, Dec.12, 1986

[33] Hood, LE, American Journal Nursing, p.459, Apr.1987

[34] Dollinger, M., EVERYONE'S GUIDE TO CANCER THERAPY, p.2, Somerville, Kansas City, 1990

[35] Grant, JP, Nutrition, vol.6, no.4, p.6S, July 1990 supl

[36] Hoffman, EJ, CANCER AND THE SEARCH FOR SELECTIVE BIOCHEMICAL INHIBITORS, CRC Press, Boca Raton, FL, 1999

KEY 1
UNDERSTAND THE PROBLEM

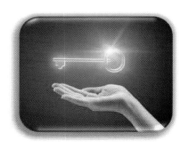

Chapter 1.1
If This Stuff Works...
Then Why Doesn't My Doctor Prescribe It
And My Insurance Company Pay For It

"Unless we put medical freedom in the constitution, the time will come when medicine will organize an undercover dictatorship."
Dr. Benjamin Rush, signer of the Declaration of Independence, 1776

This chapter is a necessary "reality orientation" in this book. This book is about healing, wholeness, optimism, empowerment, and more. Our beat is health, not business or politics. Yet, there is a lot of politics and business in our $3.5 trillion/year medical industrial complex. And the answers to the above questions may surprise or anger you.

FROM NATURE'S PHARMACY: Cruciferous Vegetables

DIM from cruciferous vegetables. In the 1950s, researchers gave two different types of diets to rats, then exposed them to radioactivity, as if they were near a nuclear blast. The rats who ate beets had a higher incidence of cancer than the rats who ate broccoli, so the researchers concluded that something in beets makes radioactivity more toxic. Two decades later, Lee Wattenberg, MD of the University of Minnesota discovered the truth regarding this previous study: there are compounds in broccoli that reduce the toxicity of radioactivity and other cancer-causing agents. The enlightened era of chemo-prevention was born. Scientists have isolated various indoles in cruciferous vegetables (broccoli, Brussels sprout, 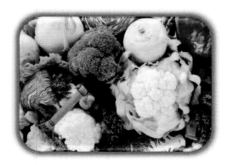 cabbage, kale, cauliflower, etc.). DIM (diindolylmethane) is one of the more promising phytonutrients that may help to reduce the damaging effects of toxins, including excess estrogens in the body. Although DIM and indoles are not considered essential nutrients, yet, they are quite valuable if you are interested in lowering your cancer risk and improving general health.

The Good News

Modern medicine. Make no mistake about it, health care in the developed countries is a glamorous show of high tech wizardry, micro robotic surgery, 3 D printing of replacement body parts, targeted drugs, gene therapy, and more. If you are in a car accident, then head straight to the nearest big city emergency room and you will get the finest care humanity has ever seen. Pain management is a major improvement over the millions of people who have died or suffered in pain without modern analgesics. Diagnostics and symptom management have evolved to an extraordinary level.

The Bad News

, Yet, Christiaan Barnard, MD, the world's first heart transplant surgeon, was asked of the greatest medical advances in human health in the past 500 years. His answer: the invention of the indoor flushing toilet, invented by John Herrington in 1596, but made widely available by Sir John Crapper in England around 1880. Toilets took away one of the primary sources of pandemic plagues: fecal to oral infections. Next on the list for major medical advances is the refrigerator, which allowed humanity to have fresh produce available nearly year around. Fruits and vegetables are a preventive and curative medicine that no drug can duplicate.

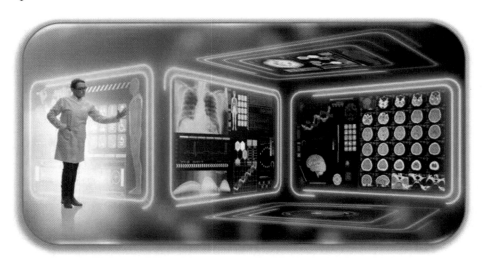

Cancer, once a rare condition found in 1% of the population, will now be diagnosed in 42% of Americans in their lifetime. Auto-immune disorders, like multiple sclerosis and rheumatoid arthritis, once found in less than 1% of the population, now affects 16% of Americans. Alzheimer's, once a rare condition, now affects 5.4 million Americans and devastates many more families when grandpa cannot remember any of his family members. 29,000 Americans died last year from the abuse of prescription opioids. Yet 4 times that many, or 128,000 died from the on label use of prescription drugs.

HEALTH STATE OF THE UNION
AMERICA NEAR THE ABYSS?

US #1 WORLD HEALTH EXPENSES $3.5 trillion/year, 50%+ 2nd
IATROGENIC DEATHS: 100,000-780,000/yr
METABOLIC DISEASE: 88% of Americans
AUTOIMMUNE DISEASE: 50 million US
US #37 HEALTH CARE SYSTEM, according to World Health Org.
HEART DISEASE: 50% of deaths, more ER, RX, disability
CANCER: #1 cause death in US; from 3% of deaths in 1900 to 24% in 1999; 42% of
Americans will develop cancer in lifetime, 8 mil treated, another 7 mil "in
remission", 250%^ br.ca. 1950
DIABETES: 30 million in US, +30 mil prediabetic, 1/3 US get DB
MIND DRUGS: 338 mil RX for depression
MEDICATION: 3rd-5th cause death US; 140,000/yr, 9.6 mil rxn/yr
OBESITY: 60% US, 300% ^ morbid OB since 1980, 90% type 2 DB
ASPIRIN: 55 billion per year in US
ALZHEIMER'S: 5.5 mil US, 14 mil 2050, 4th leading cause death US
HYPERTENSION: 60 million in US, RX increases risk for heart att.
INFECTIONS: from obscure to 3rd cause death, drug resistant strains

Medical errors kill at least <u>250,000 Americans</u> annually. Americans consume 60 million pounds of antibiotics annually, with about <u>half being fed to animals</u> for faster growth and to keep them alive in horrific conditions. Of the <u>154 million prescriptions for antibiotics</u> each year, at least 30% are inappropriate. Antibiotic use has been reckless and unrestrained, bringing about new drug resistant pathogens and the much feared MRSA. Distributing antibiotics like Halloween candy not only wreaks havoc on the microbiome of the human gut, but also creates the potential for generating a pandemic plague with drug resistant bacteria. With 70% of Americans on some prescription drug, the <u>$446 billion per year drug industry</u> now controls much of the media, Congress, and FDA. Although 15 bills have been introduced to help lower the cost of drugs to Americans, none have made it to the Senate floor, due to the <u>$240 million spent on lobbying</u> by drug companies.

2/3 of Americans are overweight, which brings with it a major increase in the risk for many diseases. 29 million Americans have diabetes with another 70 million having prediabetes, or just on the edge. Diabetes incidence has doubled in 20 years. Diabetes threatens the eyes, kidneys, nerves, brain, and blood vessels of these patients. There are 2.4 million unnecessary surgeries performed annually in the US resulting in 12,000 deaths. While America spends more than twice the amount per person on health care compared to any other country, a report from the World Health Organization ranked the US 37th out of 191 countries for the general health of the people.

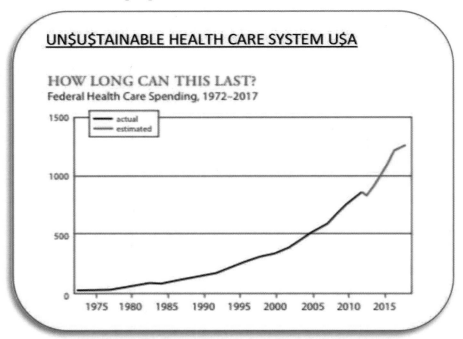

America spends twice the amount per capita on health care compared to nations that provide free healthcare for all. While some political activists want to provide free health care for all illegal aliens, health care costs are the primary cause of bankruptcy in America for working citizens. We spend 17% of our GDP on health care, with the results being 42% will get cancer, 30 million are diabetic, 2/3 are overweight, 88% have some metabolic disease, and on. According to the Institute of Medicine, 30% of our health care expenditures goes to unnecessary or counterproductive procedures, fraud, and excessive administrative costs.

How Old?

When Jesus was crucified at age 30 something, around 36 AD, he would have been an old man and at the upper limit of lifespan for those days. Average lifespan in America has increased from 45 in 1900 to 77 in 2016. Critics of this warm and fuzzy number point out that if you factor out the common plagues that afflicted many populations, especially children, then life expectancy has increased very little. Hippocrates, the father of modern medicine, died at age 90 in 370 BC. Michelangelo, crafter of some of the finest art the world has ever seen, died at age 88 in 1564 AD. Benjamin Franklin, one of the founding fathers of America, died at age 84 in 1790. The point is, people who survived the gauntlet of accidents and diseases that kill many young people, then making it to 80 becomes more likely, even without modern medicine.

Underlying Cause of Disease?

No one with a headache is suffering from a deficiency of aspirin. And no one with breast cancer is suffering from a deficiency of Perjeta and Herceptin, which costs $115,000 per year according to the manufacturer Genentech. While drugs and surgery can sometimes temporarily manage the symptoms of illness, these therapies do nothing to change the underlying cause of the disease.

What if I slammed my thumb in the desk drawer at my office every day for a week. By Friday, my thumb is black and blue, red, and swollen, painful, and bleeding. I go to Dr. A who prescribes pain medication. Dr. B prescribes corticosteroids to reduce the swelling. Dr. C recommends that we excise/remove the thumb because it looks defective. The real answer here is "stop slamming your thumb in the desk drawer." The "slamming" is the underlying cause of disease, or etiology, which is essentially ignored in modern medicine in favor of subduing symptoms with drugs.

Most "doc in the box" medicine today is 3-7 minutes with the patient, make a diagnosis, write a prescription, and move on to the next patient. Here are a few examples of this "slamming" going on widely in modern society. People eat too often, which generates insulin resistance and chronic hyperglycemia, which creates excessive fat storage, which generates elevated fats in the blood, which causes stickiness of blood cells, which creates heart disease and stroke. You can provide several expensive and dangerous drugs to treat the symptoms, or instruct the patient on intermittent fasting to eliminate the whole problem. The drug companies and junk food industry is not going to promote such effective and free therapies as fasting.

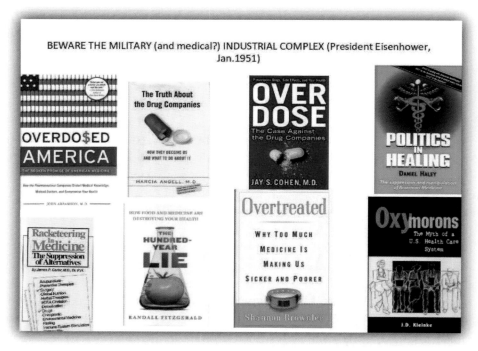

There are many very bright experts who have detailed exquisitely the dramatic advantages in using lifestyle changes (i.e. diet & exercise) over drugs. Professor of Medicine at Harvard, John Abramson, MD.

<u>Overdosed America: The Broken Promise of American Medicine</u>
The former editor of the New England Journal of Medicine, Marcia Angell, MD speaks of the disinformation and corruption in the drug industry.

<u>The Truth About the Drug Companies</u>
Ottis Brawley, MD, former scientific director for the American Cancer Society speaks of the conflict of interest in medicine where doctors choose therapies that will benefit the doctor, rather than therapies that will benefit the patient.

<u>How We Do Harm</u>
There are dozens more books like the above which document the serious problems, corruption, monopolies, control of media that makes health care in America actually sickness management.

"The only true blood sport in America is high level politics."
Hunter Thompson

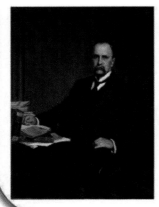

"The first duties of the physician is to educate the masses not to take medicine."

Sir William Osler, MD

1849-1919

founder of modern medicine

founder of Johns Hopkins Med. School

founder of psychosomatic medicine

Follow the Money Trail

Pure as the driven profit? The current Gross Domestic Product in America is just below $20 trillion. The federal budget of 2020 is $4.8 trillion. Health care in America is a $3.5 trillion per year business, which is over $10,000 per person and 18% of the gross domestic product. The $446 billion US pharmaceutical industry marks up their cost 50-500 fold for predatory profit margins. This is a lot of money to fight over. Special interest groups hire well positioned lobbyists to sell their agenda in Congress. Let's make prescription drugs the only real reimbursable medicine in American, put everyone else in jail or label them "quacks", then get the government to pay for the drugs so the poor bloated consumer has no out of pocket expenses. And we will get the government to pay for drug development. What a deal!

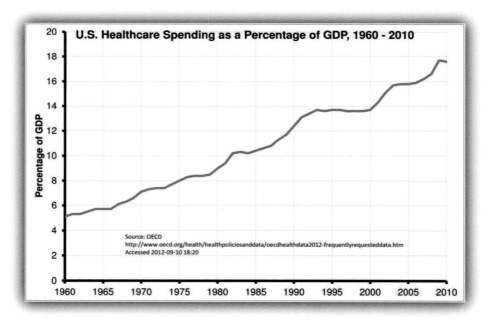

While we would all like to think that health care should be a sacred ground of humanitarian kindness with full access on a non-profit basis for all, in fact greed, profit and market share do play a significant role in health care.   At the risk of sounding gloomy, you are only worth something to this medical industrial complex if you are halfway between well and dead.

"Where large sums of money are concerned, it is advisable to trust nobody."
Agatha Christie

Most of the one million medical doctors in America are bright and caring people who want to make a difference in the lives of their patients. However, these doctors are trained in medical schools where nutrition is ignored and even ridiculed. Pharmaceuticals and surgery are the real medicine, plus some radiation, targeted immune therapies and some obscure DNA therapy spin offs. Everything else is "alternative medicine" or quackery. Most of these alternatives are not insurance reimbursable. Most Americans are heavily or completely dependent on their health insurance provider. If the therapy is not covered by the insurance company, then they cannot or will not pay for it. Hence, the true gatekeeper here is the question "what therapies are insurance reimbursable?"

The Gatekeeper
The International Code of Diseases (ICD-10) contains over 70,000 codes for specific diagnoses of diseases. The World Health Organization creates this massive online database, and from this database comes the "cookbook" medicine which the doctor must follow as "standard of care"...which, of course, is controlled by the pharmaceutical industry. Once the diagnosis is made, the only protocol acceptable, if you want to keep your medical license, is to follow the drugs and surgery approach to medicine. Hence, all other therapies are non-reimbursable, or possibly subject to criminal prosecution.

Self-Reliant vs. Dependent
While America was founded on the principles of freedom, privacy, and personal accountability; those values seem to have morphed into a nation of dependent and entitled people. The average American is heavily

in debt. The average American dies owing $62,000. 68% of people die owing money on their credit cards.

Immediate gratification

One might be tempted to point the finger of blame entirely at the drug companies. Yet many Americans want to eat, drink, smoke, think, and do anything they want…then head to the doctor for drugs to subdue the inevitable consequences of an unhealthy life. Americans want immediate gratification and the drug companies and junk food industry are eager to sell them what they want.

Around 1970 Stanford professor Walter Mischel conducted a series of experiments on pre-school children in which the children were offered a marshmallow now, or if the child could wait 15 minutes, then they would get 2 marshmallows. About 1/3 of the children had the stamina to wait 15 minutes for the second marshmallow, called the "waiters". About 1/3 of the children grabbed the marshmallow immediately and couldn't wait. About 1/3 of the children waited a few minutes, then realized they could not last 15 minutes and took the one marshmallow. Hence, 2/3 of the children were "grabbers", or 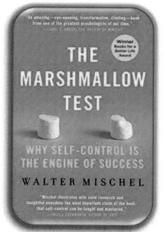 sought immediate gratification. All of this data would have become meaningless trivia were it not for the fact that Professor Mischel's daughter was one of the subjects in the original study. About 15 years after the study, Mischel's daughter told her father "Dad, seems like the grabbers are having more problems in life, while the waiters are doing better in careers, relationships, with their health, etc.

So here is the crux of the problem. 2/3 of Americans are overweight. 70% of Americans are using prescription medications to palliate symptoms. 80% of Americans are in debt. 70% of Americans admit to little or no exercise. Do you see a trend? The $446 billion US pharmaceutical industry spent $5.2 billion per year on direct to consumer ads. The primary advertiser on TV is drug companies. Do you think they will allow news stories on the superiority of lifestyle changes vs. drug use?

WHAT PRESCRIPTION DRUGS REALLY COST				
BRAND NAME®	DOSAGE	PRICE $/ 100 CAPS	COST $ GENERIC ACTIVE INGREDIENT	PERCENT MARKUP
Celebrex	100 mg	$130.27	$0.60	21,612%
Claritin	10 mg	215.17	0.71	30,206
Keflex	250 mg	157.39	1.88	8,272
Lipitor	20 mg	272.37	5.80	4,596
Norvasc	10 mg	188.29	0.14	134,393
Prevacid	30 mg	344.77	1.01	34,036
Prilosec	20 mg	419.00	0.52	80,477
Prozac	20 mg	247.47	0.11	224,873
Tenormin	50 mg	104.47	0.13	80,262
Vasotec	10 mg	102.37	0.20	51,085
Xanax	1 mg	136.79	0.02	569,858
Zoloft	50 mg	206.87	1.75	11,721
Source: Life Extension Magazine, Mar.2005, p.11				

Human cravings

The human tongue has four primary sensors: sour, sweet, salt, and bitter. Hot peppers affect the pain sensors, hence none of the above. The fast food industry (i.e. McDonalds) earns $200 billion per year in revenue, which does not begin to include the soft drink industry, sugar breakfast cereals, and other foods that are for instant gratification, but not for nourishing the human body. The food industry employs thousands of food scientists who know more about your food cravings than do you. They conduct experiments and focus groups, and know how to put the "hook in the lip" of the customer. You may not know

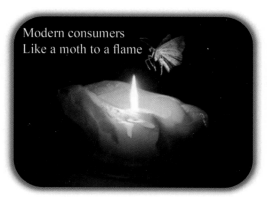

Modern consumers
Like a moth to a flame

it, but many junk food customers are like a moth to a flame, enticed by the flame but will soon be destroyed by the flame.

Safety Net vs Hammock

We are all in favor of helping people who cannot help themselves. The slippery slope here is helping people who can help themselves and turning their "safety net" into a hammock. At that point we hear the words of the cynic: "No good deed goes unpunished." Americans have been lulled into a sense of complacence about health and lifestyle habits. Immediate gratification turns into chronic drug use, which eventually leads to some really serious disease for which drugs and surgery are impotent, like most of the 50 million Americans suffering from the 100 different auto-immune conditions, or stage four any cancer. 100 million Americans have eaten themselves into medical obesity with a Pandora's box of ailments attached. Should we pay for the healthcare required from this semi-suicidal lifestyle?

Medical Myopia
"What you are not up on, you are down on."

Doctors are far more likely to suffer license revocation for using "non-standard care", aka nutrition therapy, than if that doctor was guilty of malpractice, excessive prescriptions for patients, or even molesting a patient. While nutrition therapy is a well-developed science, modern medicine and the government "protective agencies" spend considerable time prosecuting and discouraging the practice of nutrition therapy. There are numerous well-referenced textbooks on nutritional medicine, including <u>Alan Gaby, MD Nutritional Medicine</u> with over 1300 pages and 15,000 references. The debate over the legitimacy of nutritional medicine is over.

Government and Health

But don't my elected representatives have my best interests? Under the guise of helping the people, politicians ask for votes on the basis of "we are going to do something about_____ (fill in the blank for the disease)". The federal government spends about $980 billion/yr on health care, including $527 billion on Medicare, $352 billion on Medicaid and State Children's Health Insurance Program, $61 billion for Veteran's, $41 billion for subsidies for uninsured people, etc. Medicare Part D, which was started in 2006 to assist seniors in acquiring their prescription drugs, now costs over $100 billion/yr. And, by law, the <u>federal government is not allowed to negotiate</u> the price of the drugs. Imagine buying over $100 billion worth of anything each year and you pay retail price, no volume discounts. Your Congress hard at work on your behalf.

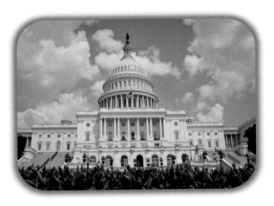

But that does not count the research arm of the federal government. The National Institutes of Health has a $37 billion per budget that mostly funds 50,000 research projects orchestrated by 300,000 researchers at 2500 universities. Nearly all of that money is spent on basic research (trying to understand nature and the human body) or drug research. The <u>National Library of Medicine</u> catalogs over 28 million scientific studies which can be accessed on the internet. You can also access scientific records via <u>Google scholar</u>, which helps the consumer to become better informed on their own health. Using these sources, you can see how legitimate this field of nutrition has become. Unless…

Most health experts agree that excess sugar in our diet is killing us.[1] When the Food and Nutrition Board as part of the Institute of Medicine, an advisory branch of Congress, attempted to recommend lowering the amount of sugar in our diet, the sugar industry lobbied vigorously to cut Congressional funding to the World Health Organization. We currently get about 20% of our calories from sugar. The new recommendation is that we should get no more than 25% of our calories from sugar. That's right. Eat more sugar with the endorsement of the experts, who are hamstrung by the lobbyists who are controlled by the invisible puppeteers in our economy.

Control information.

"By means of shrewd lies, unremittingly repeated, it is possible to make people believe that heaven is hell, and hell heaven. The greater the lie, the more readily it will be believed."
Adolph Hitler, 1936

When Adolph Hitler took control of Germany in 1933, the Nazi party controlled only 3% of the country's 4700 newspapers. Within months, a Propaganda Ministry was initiated to eliminate any news "calculated to weaken the strength of the Reich abroad or at home." No dissenting opinions were allowed. Legitimate reporters and radio broadcasters disappeared. Hitler convinced one of the most accomplished people on earth, who dominated science, medicine, art, and music to follow an insane path…all because Hitler controlled the minds of the people through the media.

A similar struggle for the control of information is occurring throughout the world. North Korea, Iran, and other totalitarian regimes heavily control access to the internet and thoroughly "sanitize" the news before anyone gets to see it. A colossal battle is being waged in the US for control of information. Google, Facebook, Twitter, Wikipedia, and YouTube among others, constantly "edit" sites or content that they feel is unacceptable. "Deplatforming" or being banned for conservative views has become rampant by the tech giants. Search <u>Johanna Budwig on Wikipedia</u> and you find a ridiculous statement: "There is no evidence that this or other <u>"anti-cancer" diet</u> is effective." Which is blatantly untrue.

Big Pharma knows the power of controlling the media and the tech giants on the internet. They then control the minds of the people. No matter who you voted for in the presidential election of 2016, you must admit the media has lost interest in "objective journalism" and merely spins their highly skewed perspective to the public.

Mandatory Vaccinations?

Of the $1 trillion/yr global pharmaceutical business, about $60 billion comes from vaccines, with about half of that based in the USA. Vaccine proponents say the vaccine issue is settled. However, there is compelling evidence that vaccines are <u>neither safe nor effective</u>, and given that argument, they should certainly not be mandatory. There is a 500 page compilation of 1200 peer reviewed studies showing the risks found in our current vaccine schedule of 26 shots by age 2. The incidence of autism and developmental delays has skyrocketed from 1 in 5000 in 1975 to 1 in 59 today, possibly due to our vaccination schedule.

Vaccine manufacturers are immune from lawsuits if harm is done. By 1986, there had been so many personal injury lawsuits filed against vaccine manufacturers that the federal government passed the <u>National Childhood Vaccine Injury Act of 1986</u> to exempt vaccine manufacturers from harm. Soon thereafter, the <u>Vaccine Adverse Events Reporting System</u> was launched to allow people to report problems from vaccines. According to this system, the few people who actually enter their data, 436 children

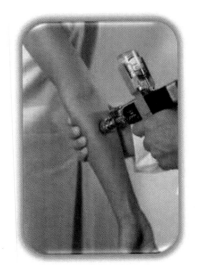

died from vaccines in 2016. This is a long way from "safe".

Insurance or the government pays for the vaccinations, so the patient has no out of pocket expense. States like California mandate vaccines before a child can enter school. No exceptions. Vaccine information about hazards are scrubbed from the web. "Anti-vaxxers" are deplatformed from the web. No dissenting voices will be heard, although there are many articulate and science-based arguments against our aggressive vaccination program, such as The Truth About Vaccines. We need an intelligent discussion about the risk/benefit/cost of vaccines, then drop the legal mandate. Laws take away freedoms. If the vaccines work, then you should not be concerned that someone else does not take the vaccine. Mankind survived this long without vaccines, and primarily due to healthy immune systems generated by breastfeeding, a whole food diet, healthy guts, and quarantines, or placing blatantly sick people in a safe zone away from the healthy masses.

If You Can't Beat Them, Then Deceive Them

The spin zone. Spin is a means of propaganda, of twisting information to make your story look better than it should. Throughout the dark ages in Europe (550-1400 AD) the Catholic Church had an iron fist on the people and politics. Any actions that annoyed the Church were ruled as heresy, blasphemy, apostasy, and often the perpetrator was condemned to death. Galileo, the inventor of the first telescope and first real astronomer, was put under house arrest for the duration of his life for a discovery that would have earned him world fame today.

Fast forward to the 1950s where Senator Joseph McCarthy (1908-1957) held hearings in Congress accusing nearly everyone of being a communist sympathizer, or comm symp. Many innocent people had their lives and careers destroyed by this insane campaign. Fast forward to 2018 where anyone who did not agree with a certain group of people was labelled a "fascist" or "racist". Most of the time these labels were totally inappropriate, but served the purpose of the attacker with propaganda, or the "spin".

Since the 1960s Big Pharma has controlled the media through advertising dollars and lobbyists to attack anyone who dared to stray from the party line of drugs and surgery for any condition. These heretics or comm symps or fascists were called "quacks", using "pseudo-science" or "junk science" or "charlatans". All of these labels were intended to discredit the physicians who were using their 12 years of training to help patients.

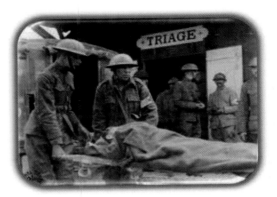

Triage

Coming from a French word meaning "separate, sift, select", triage in health care was originated during the Napoleanic wars in Europe in the early 19th century. Combat surgeons would select which wounded soldier could receive the most beneficial care. You might have 50 soldiers with minor wounds that could be patched up in the same time that one might spend trying the save the life of one seriously wounded soldier. The term is unpopular among some, yet essential when people realize that no one has unlimited money and time to address every health care. Over half of all health expenses are spent on 5% of all patients.

"but you're still gonna die" Song by Shel Silverstein

Over 40% of Medicare expenses are for people in their last month of life. In other words, the medical intervention made no difference. Doctors see jousting with death as a titanic battle for dominance of intellect and technology. Patients cling to each precious second of life, knowing someone else is paying for what might be a losing cause. Everyone wants grandma to die somewhere else, certainly not at home. Our ancestors embraced the circle of life. Young people would watch grandma die at home and know that she was with loved ones, and that each of us gets a turn at death, hopefully with dignity. More on "you're still gonna die" in the chapter on Mind.

It Takes Two to Dance

Where did this bizarre "dance" of healthcare originate? Junk food and medicine constitute a huge percentage of the GDP. More money was spent on <u>soft drinks than any other food category</u> in America. The people want to believe that they can eat, drink, smoke, think, and do anything they want and modern medicine will fix the inevitable consequences of that unhealthy lifestyle. And someone else will pay for it. Drug companies feed on this natural tendency of immediate gratification of the public. And then it gets worse.

Protecting the Public?

Whistleblowers, like <u>Dr. David Graham,</u> associate director of the Food and Drug Administration office of drug safety testified in Congress in 2005 saying:

"FDA is inherently biased in favor of the pharmaceutical industry. It views industry as its client, whose interests it must represent and advance. It views its primary mission as approving as many drugs it can, regardless of whether the drugs are safe or needed."

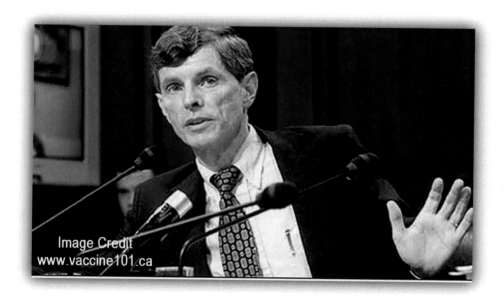

Image Credit
www.vaccine101.ca

Dr. Graham earned his Medical Degree and Masters in Public Health and sacrificed his career at the FDA in testifying. His courage and intelligence needs to be heeded.

And nothing changed about the system of healthcare management, drug advertising, monitoring adverse drug events, etc. Vioxx was a painkiller drug used from 1999-2004 which probably caused the premature deaths of 500,000 people. And no one associated with this catastrophe saw the inside of a courtroom. The sheriff is owned by the biggest ranchers in the valley. Meaning, the various government agencies that are entrusted with protecting the public have become infested with the industries they are supposed to regulate. The fox is guarding the chicken coop.

Suggestion

Let's keep the FDA, yet take away its prosecutorial powers. There are already many laws in place that allow for legal action in case of personal injury. Let's use the awesome power of the internet to make or break practitioners, products, procedures, etc. eBay and Amazon are among the pioneers of developing legitimate rating systems. You cannot review a product unless you bought it. Add all of these reviews and you have a much better system for purging the marketplace of useless or dangerous products and professionals. FDA would be like Underwriter's Laboratory, or UL. If people find that having the UL seal is meaningful, then UL becomes a badge of merit on the product. If FDA endorsement on the product does not constitute safety or efficacy, then people will ignore it or reject it. Let the free marketplace decide what stays and what goes. Put the incompetent practitioners and products out of business.

What Does It Cost?

Who cares? In March of 2017 your author was doing stretches, not unlike the splits. Felt like a cold knife stabbing me in the gut. Days later, the knife wound vacillated between icy and hot. Days later I reasoned that I needed more stretching, more splits. Eventually I went to a doctor who diagnosed an inguinal hernia. The snake had poked through the pillow case. Eventually, I went to a surgeon who recommended surgery. I asked what this procedure costs. No one knew. Not the doctor, nor the director of billing in this mega- surgery empire. It took 3 days of fact-gathering for the financial director of this surgery suite to inform me that my co-pay was "around $1000". I asked, what does the procedure cost, in total. No one knew. No one cared. Let the insurance company and the biller fight it out.

We have detached the most fundamental link in capitalism: the buyer from the seller. The buyer should be the patient. The seller should be the surgeon. Neither had anything to do with this transaction. That is asking for trouble. More on my non-surgical recovery from inguinal hernia later.

Yes, there is an ICD (international code of diseases) 10 version of what is the exact differential diagnosis and what is reimbursable. Yet, the point is, we have made a mockery out of the capitalistic system. Adam Smith, around the signing of the Declaration of Independence, argued that free market competition will provide the best service or product at the best price. And he has been proven correct in many instances. In 1982 the federally protected monopoly of AT&T was considered a monopoly by a federal judge, which began the biggest dispersion of a corporation in history. In 1984 it cost $72 (accounting for inflation) for a 30 minute phone call from US to Europe. Today you can make unlimited phone calls from your cell phone around the US and using cell phone apps (like Skype) you can call anywhere in the world for $0.02/minute. That is the benefit of free market competition.

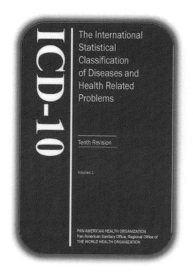

Same thing happened in the medical industry, where allowed. Most areas of medicine are heavily controlled by government and the insurance industry. However, plastic surgery, i.e. elective surgery is not reimbursable. Costs have plummeted while quality has increased dramatically due to the influences of a free market system

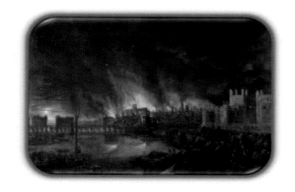

Insurance

In 1666, the most prestigious city on earth, London, was devastated by a fire. The local merchants gathered together to structure "shared risk" in the first effort at insurance. You could not buy fire insurance from this pool of merchants unless you complied with numerous standards, i.e. you want to prevent a fire. You would not insure a burning building. You would not provide fire insurance for a smoking drunk who liked to throw tequila on his fireplace. That is where health insurance loses contact with reality. Insurance actuaries are statistical geniuses who crunch numbers to protect their employers. Insurance is essentially a bet. Insurance companies are in the business of making money. Nothing wrong with that. Health insurance has deviated so far from actuary science as to be ludicrous.

Unrealistic Expectations

Some people want to get something for nothing. They want Santa Claus to bring them everything. They want their action heroes (Tarzan, Superman, Batman, etc.) to save them. And if no one will save me, then I will sue someone. In 1990 the Americans with Disabilities Act (ADA) was passed, allegedly to help the 2 million people in wheelchairs and others with legitimate handicaps. Instead, conditions like obesity have become a feeding trough for lawyers. Obesity, which is self-inflicted from poor lifestyle choices, is very different than someone in a wheelchair from multiple sclerosis. Obesity, as defined by 100% above normal weight, is considered a disability, like cancer or blindness.

We need to expect to pay something for our health care. People confuse "freeways" with "tollways". No road was free to build, you just paid for it through taxes. No health care is free, you just pay for it through taxes or added costs on our purchases. Someone paid for it. People who spend much of their time setting their hair on fire (unhealthy lifestyle) need to suffer the consequences or pay the cost of repair.

Risk vs Benefits vs Costs

Nearly all business decisions involve juggling the components of risk, benefit, and cost. Not so in health care. While health insurance companies will not pay for nutrition consultations, they will pay for the $3000 per day spent in the hospital once the patient becomes malnourished. Few insurance companies will pay for nutrition supplements, yet all will pay $13,700 per year in medical bills for the routine diabetic care or $70,000 to $200,000 for heart bypass surgery. While most doctors are not allowed to profit from the prescribing and sale of a drug, oncologists are the exception to the rule. "Buy and bill" provides the majority of an oncologist's income. And its these people who are most strident against the use of nutritional medicine. All of which quite probably could have been prevented by using lifestyle medicine, integrative medicine, nutritional medicine, functional medicine, pragmatic medicine…call it what you will.

Is Chemo Effective?

When examining risk to benefit to cost ratio of chemo for cancer patients, we find that the side effects for most chemo drugs as listed on the Mayo Clinic website include: damage to heart, lungs, kidneys, nerves (causing painful neuropathy), inducing cancer, and the routine nausea, vomiting, hair loss, fever, loss of appetite, bruising, immune suppression, and more. So the risks are high. What are the benefits? There have been many studies showing the relative ineffectiveness of chemo in treating cancer. One of the more respected published article showed that chemo works in about 2% of all cancer patients. Yet chemo is given to nearly 2/3 of cancer patients. And chemo may even cause the cancer to spread or metastasize.

Does Nutrition Neutralize the "Effectiveness" of Chemo?

No. <u>Beyond argument.</u> Hundreds of studies have been conducted with the overwhelming consensus that nutrition support minimizes the damage of the chemo to the patient, thus sparing the patient unnecessary side effects (like painful neuropathy) and potential cancers down the road, while never reducing the "effectiveness" of chemo. <u>Nutrition makes chemo and radiation</u> more of a targeted weapon against the cancer, rather than a general toxin against both the patient and the cancer.

Bottom Line

Let's end the government protected monopoly that Big Pharma has on the health care industry. Let the free market system decide what works. Connect the customer (patient) with the vendor (doctor or whatever). Let insurance actuaries crunch their numbers and create a legitimate cost for health insurance.

You say that people will suffer? We currently have the worst of both worlds. A health care system can be single payer, i.e. the government, or free market. The US has the worst aspects of both of those models. The most common cause of bankruptcy in America is health care

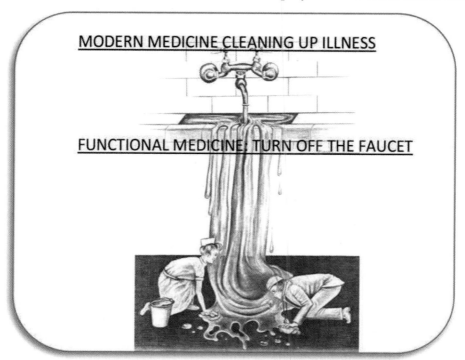

costs. The only people fully covered for any health procedure are felons in prison and illegal aliens. Am not making that up. Yes, we need charity health care. Before the Medicare act of 1965, most doctors were expected to spend 20% of their time attending to the poor. And that system worked quite well.

21st Century Medicine

What if meditation could reverse mild to moderate depression, anxiety, and insomnia without medication? What if intermittent fasting could reverse most cases of type 2 diabetes and obesity? What if a couple thousand dollars invested in lifestyle reprogramming could prevent the need for patients institutionalized with stroke or heart disease? What if a couple pennies worth of vitamin supplements could prevent and reverse many common ailments? What if a healthy lifestyle could prevent and reverse most degenerative diseases. These are not hypothetical dreams for the future. These are therapies awaiting you right now. They work. They have little or no side effects. They are dramatically cheaper than drugs and surgeries. Let the future of health care begin.

For more information on the war on cancer go to GettingHealthier.com

PATIENT PROFILE:
Ann E. Fonfa, annieappleseedpr@aol.com

I was diagnosed with breast cancer in January 1993. Because of extreme Multiple Chemical Sensitivity, I ended up refusing chemotherapy, had no radiation and no hormonal therapy. The main things I changed, was what I ate, becoming a 100% organic vegan, exercising daily for an hour, and starting on dietary supplements.

I found Dr. Quillin's book very early on thankfully. There was no Internet but a book with the exciting and satisfying title of Beating Cancer With Nutrition, meant so much to me. I even shared the information with other women in my support group who were going through conventional treatments. Some of them were brave enough to add these ideas to their own protocols and received benefits. I have always been grateful for the wisdom Dr. Quillin imparted which made me feel confident in the path I chose.

My own outcome was completely different than everyone else as I continued to have small tumors (largest was 1.5 cm). Amazingly all but the first were growing slower than normal cells and from the first recurrence onward I was told not to take chemotherapy. Eventually I met a Chinese Herbalist who prescribed an herbal protocol for me, which despite his initial request to only do his herbs, I added to my existing program. MRI-proven free of cancer in September 2001. I share all information about my protocols and evidence-based ideas on getting and staying well during treatment and after via **Annie Appleseed Project**, the all-volunteer nonprofit I founded. We also host annual conferences. 26 years after my diagnosis, I am still in remission.

ENDNOTES

[1] https://onlinelibrary.wiley.com/doi/abs/10.1111/obr.12040

KEY 2
UNDERSTAND THE SOLUTION

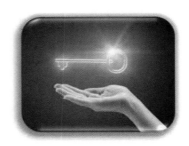

Chapter 2
How Your Body Can Fight Cancer
Under the Hood Examination of Your Body's
Innate Mechanisms for Defeating Cancer

"Illnesses do not come upon us out of the blue. They are developed from small daily sins against Nature. When enough sins have accumulated, illnesses will suddenly appear."
Hippocrates, father of modern medicine, circa 400 BC

FROM NATURE'S PHARMACY: Carrots

      Around <u>500,000 children go blind</u> each year from vitamin A deficiency.[1] Most of this occurs in Africa and Southeast Asia, where green and orange fruits and vegetables are available, but not commonly part of the diet. Beta-carotene in carrots is converted into vitamin A in the body

---

to regulate many functions, including vision. There are over 300 studies showing that a diet rich in fruits and vegetables lowers the risk for most cancers and heart disease. Carrots are the poor person's ginseng, since they are delicious, available year around, affordable, and pretty. Carrots are a rich source of beta-carotene and other carotenoids, vitamin C, pectin, potassium, K-1, B-6 and more. The <u>phytochemical soup</u> in carrots makes the drug developers green with envy.[2] Lutein, lycopenes, anthocyanins, and polyacetylenes are among the anti-oxidants and bio-regulators that are found in carrots. The glycemic index (GI) of raw carrots is very low with cooked or pureed carrots scoring higher on GI. Steamed, pressure cooked, baked, pureed, or raw…there is always room for carrots.

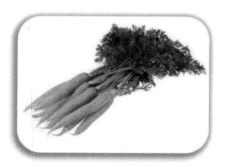

Some people shop for a new or used car based on appearance or gas mileage or performance. Some people want to look under the hood at their new car. How does it work? Feed me some impressive facts about this car's engineering and design. If you are a person who likes to know how it works, then read on. If you are less inclined toward the technical details of the human body's host defense mechanisms, then skip to the next chapter. This chapter is not a textbook for anyone, but a short summary to tempt the bright reader into better understanding the link between nutrition and cancer.

Cancer is not new to the human species or even other forms of life. The duck billed dinosaur from 70 million years ago experienced common cancers. Human skeletons from 1.7 million years ago were found with tumors. 40% of Americans born today will experience cancer in their lifetime. Cancer used to be a rare

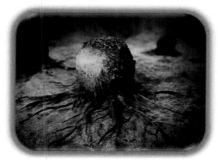

footnote among healers. That is both good news and bad news. The good news is that since cancer has been with us for eons means that we have developed numerous elegant molecular pathways for thwarting cancer. The bad news is that our current lifestyle has promoted cancer from a rare condition into the second leading cause of death in western society. Nourishing our life force is like reinstating the shell protection on an oyster with a pearl within it. Your life force is that pearl. Physical and metaphysical forces protect that life force. This book is about re-establishing your body's awesome capacity to heal itself.

DNA Integrity

You have about 37 trillion cells in your adult body. Cells are constantly dividing and dying. You generate around 240 billion new cells each day. If any of these 240 billion new cells are defective, then a quality control process begins in the human body. The cell division process involves many nutrients: folate, B-6, riboflavin, vitamin D, RNA, DNA, B-12, etc. Deficiencies of any of these methylation nutrients could lead to

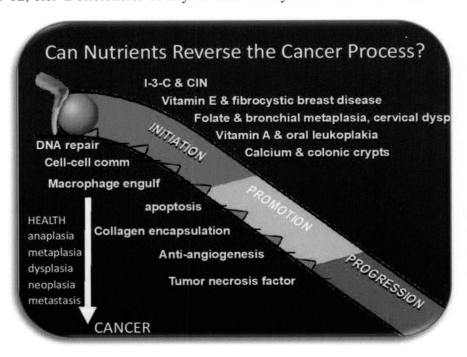

fragile DNA and defects in the newly spawned cell. Various nutrients, like vitamin A, help cells to "talk" to each other, or cell to cell communication. Deficiencies in these communication nutrients can lead to a rogue cell ignoring the call of its neighbors to "normalize or die".

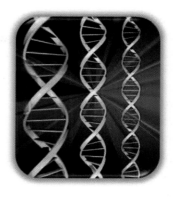

Telomeres are the ends of the DNA strands, like the plastic tips on shoelaces. Telomeres are a scoreboard for your aging process. If you are aging rapidly, then your telomeres are shorter and you are more prone to cancer. Many nutrients, including vitamins E, C, beta carotene, and omega 3 fats, <u>help to protect the telomeres from premature aging</u>.

Manipulating our Genes

Epigenetics is the science of studying how genes can be influenced by lifestyle. We are not prisoners of our genes. We do have genetic predispositions. Some diseases run in families. But 90% of our health is driven by lifestyle, which is what this book is all about. Many nutrients affect genetic expression. In one study, researchers used agouti mice that are specifically bred to develop obesity and diabetes, then gave the pregnant mice methylation nutrients (folate, B-12, etc.) and found that the <u>offspring from this bath of</u>

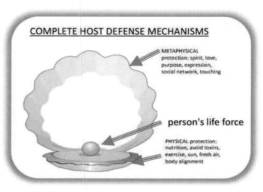

<u>methylation nutrients</u> did not develop obesity or diabetes, and even were a different color fur. Nutrition clearly affects genetic expression. A physician who inadvertently <u>discovered that he had brain cancer</u>, then spent his time researching how nutrition could enhance his outcome wrote: "The American diet is fertilizer for cancer." <u>Dr. Servan-Schreiber</u> lived

19 years after his diagnosis, which was well beyond the anticipated 1-2 year lifespan expected for his brain cancer.

Apoptosis

Cells have a life cycle, just like people. Cells are born, they mature, then age (senescence), then die, which is programmed cell death or apoptosis. Cancer cells are immortal and forget to die. There are various nutrients and food factors (vitamin E succinate, curcumin, blueberries, seaweed) to encourage apoptosis in cancer cells.

Mitochondrial Vulnerability

Mitochondria are the football shaped organelles within a cell that "burn" our food for energy. They are the energy factories. Each normal cell contains about 1000-2000 mitochondria which makes up about 20% of the cell interior. It is here that <u>Otto Warburg, MD, PhD</u> found his major breakthrough on cancer and was awarded the Nobel Prize in Medicine in 1931. Warburg was nominated 47 times throughout his career for the Nobel Prize.

Warburg found that normal cells mutate through some defect in cell respiration, beginning in the mitochondria. This defect leads the new cell to become anaerobic or more like a fermenting yeast than a healthy normal cell. PET scans use this difference in sugar vs normal metabolism by injecting the cancer patient with radioactive glucose, which is the favorite food for cancer cells, then scanning the patient's body with a Geiger counter like device to find the radioactive sugar, because that is where the cancer is…because cancer is an obligate glucose metabolizer, or sugar feeder. This defect in mitochondria can come about because of any number of flaws in nutrition, including the need for precursors of Kreb's cycle oxidation: thiamin, niacin, riboflavin, lipoic acid, etc. Acidosis, or a low (acidic) pH in the body reduces the amount of oxygen that can be absorbed by the tissue. Lacking sufficient oxygen, the cell might switch to anaerobic fuel burning just to stay alive.

AMPK

There are major metabolic pathways that are being researched for their key role in maintaining homeostasis in the human body. The body must constantly adjust its needs. Should we breakdown tissue (catabolism) or build tissue (anabolism)? Do we have enough energy to keep the orchestra of life making beautiful music? <u>AMPK is an Achilles heel of health</u>.

NUTRIENTS AS BIOLOGICAL RESPONSE MODIFIERS
changing the way the body works to reverse cancer

→IMMUNE REGULATORS, ELIMINATE INFECTIONS?
→ALTER GENETIC EXPRESSION OF CANCER
→CELL MEMBRANE DYNAMICS
→DETOXIFICATION
→PH MAINTENANCE, BALANCING PROTONS
→PROOXIDANTS & AOX, BALANCING ELECTRONS
→CELLULAR COMMUNICATIONS
→SIGNAL CELL TRANSDUCTION
→PROSTAGLANDIN REGULATION
→STEROID HORMONE CONTROL
→ENERGY METABOLISM:AEROBIC VS ANAEROBIC
→PROBIOTICS VS DYSBIOSIS
→ANTI-PROLIFERATIVE AGENTS
→ALTER TUMOR PROTECTIVE MECHANISMS
→APOPTOSIS, PROGRAMMED CELL DEATH

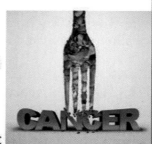

Other major metabolic pathways include sirtuins and mTOR. These pathways can be preserved in healthy mode through a variety of nutritional mechanisms: resveratrol, green tea, broccoli, etc. If these normal production lines in the cell are disturbed, then cancer and premature aging can be the result.

Essential Ingredients/Nutrients

Malnutrition is often seen as some starving baby in a third world country. In fact, malnutrition can be defined as an excess, deficiency, or imbalance of any nutrient. 92% of Americans are deficient in one or more essential nutrients, according to the United States Department of Agriculture. <u>Long term sub-clinical deficiencies</u> in any nutrient can lead to fragile DNA, which causes mutations, and the cancer cells are off to the races. Optimal nutrient intake coupled with intermittent fasting (explained later in this book) is of paramount importance in preventing and reversing cancer.

Hale Project

In a study of 1500 men and women ages 70-90 in 11 countries in Europe, researchers found that people who followed the Mediterranean diet, did not smoke, consumed moderate amounts of alcohol, and exercised, had a 50% reduction in all-cause mortality. If this healthy lifestyle were a drug, it would be headline news around the world. No prescription required and it's free.

Immune Protection

If that rogue cell begins to duplicate, then the immune system is called in. Immune cells, like natural killer cells and macrophages, are trained to recognize the difference between "self and non-self" and then destroy the invader. Sometimes the cancer invader sets up a stealth barrier using a shield as if the cancer pod were a fetus, thus escaping the recognition of the immune warriors. Proteolytic enzymes help to erode the stealth barrier from the cancer so the immune system can recognize

and eliminate it. There have been very promising results using nutrition supplements consisting of numerous digestive enzymes to slow cancer growth. When we eat whole live raw food, like fruits and vegetables, we consume small amounts of live enzymes, of which some will pass through the intestinal lining into the bloodstream.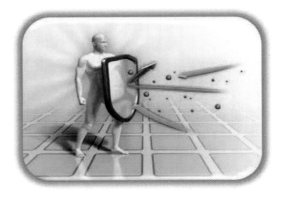

There are numerous mechanisms that have been proposed to explain why a diet rich in vegetables absolutely lowers the risk for most cancers.

Angiogenesis

If the cancer rogue continues to grow, then it will need a blood supply to bring in nutrients and expel waste products. Making new blood vessels (angiogenesis) is critical for the growth of a tumor. There are various nutrients (like EPA from fish oil) and food extracts (like cartilage and seaweed) that help to shut down the making of blood vessels from a tumor. Nutrients including vitamin C, lysine, proline, and green tea have shown promise in <u>shutting down angiogenesis from tumors</u>.

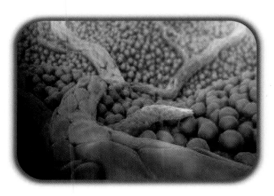

Collagen Encapsulation

If the cancer has now become a measurable tumor, then the body will try to wall off the cancer with a thick covering of calcium and collagen. Tumor encapsulation is the next phase of "damage control" in the human body. This <u>extremely important and complex process</u> appears to be a war between the host body trying to wall off the tumor and the tumor generating enzymes to pierce the collagen envelope.

Inflammation

Many experts teach that cancer is the inevitable consequence of long-term inflammation. Inflammation is when the body is responding to an insult, a toxin, a food that induces swelling (like sugar or omega 6 oils). C reactive protein is a useful marker in the blood for measurable inflammation. Many components in a healthy diet are designed to reduce inflammation: fruits, vegetables, polyphenols, turmeric, fish oil, bioflavonoids, carotenoids, etc.

Glycation

Glycation is the process whereby glucose/sugar in the blood gets attached to various proteins and DNA, then causes a reaction that "cooks" (cross linkage) the body. End stage diabetes is a glaring example of too much glycation or cooking of the body parts: kidney failure, gangrene and amputation of limbs, hardening and blockage of the smaller blood vessels, blindness, cognitive decline, etc. Diabetes increases the risk for most cancers by 50-100%. All of glycation can be controlled through diet, avoiding the wrong foods, including the right foods, exercise, stress reduction, the right supplements, and regular intermittent fasting.

Oxidation

Oxidation is the process of "rusting" within. We need oxygen to live. We also generate free radicals from this aerobic process that cause a deterioration of everything from DNA to the immune soldiers. Slowing the oxidation process is key to preventing and reversing cancer. While the oncologist seeks to utilize free radicals through chemo and radiation, the body's inherent anti-cancer mechanisms are fed by antioxidants, such as found in whole plant food and many medicinal spices. In fact, providing antioxidants to the cancer patient while the oncologist uses pro-oxidants has been shown to be a synergistic benefit.

Detoxification

We generate toxins as a normal by-product of living. We also consume toxins in our air, food, and water supply. We also generate toxins within the gut when dysbiosis or the unfriendly microbes control the gut, aka endotoxemia. Toxins include heavy metals (lead, mercury, cadmium, aluminum, arsenic) and by-products of the petroleum industry, persistent organic pollutants that are at scary levels in modern society.[3] Toxins create havoc with our delicate DNA, our fragile hormone balance, our immune system, the brain, developing fetus, and much more. We need to clean up our act or our cancer epidemic will be with us for the foreseeable future. More on this in the chapter on detoxification.

A HEALTHY HUMAN BODY IS SELF-REGULATING AND SELF-REPAIRING

REMOVE BLOCKS	PROVIDE
ie toxins	essential nutrients
stress	psycho spiritual
EMF	exercise
infections	energy alignment

A well-nourished cancer patient can better manage the disease.

Your Game Plan

Your body works wonders every day, but only if you do your part. The components of health that keep your body in healthy condition include:

- ✓ Attitude
- ✓ Nutrition
- ✓ Exercise
- ✓ Toxins
- ✓ Energy alignment
- ✓ Microbiome

Each of these vectors will be discussed in some detail throughout this book. No one said that getting healthier was easy. But it is mandatory that you do your part in your healing process.

For more information on how your body can fight cancer go to GettingHealthier.com

PATIENT PROFILE

J.B. was diagnosed with stage 4 prostate cancer in 2010. He underwent surgery, radiation and other treatments recommended by his Oncologist, but none of it worked. He says, "My doctors were killing me. My Oncologist and Urologist kept giving me more drugs, I was feeling bad, there was pain. I did not want to live like a human skeleton living in a wheelchair." He heard Dr. Quillin at <u>The Truth About Cancer</u> and read Beating Cancer with Nutrition. J.B. resonated with what PQ had to say. He had an initial phone consultation with PQ late 2015. J.B. keeps Beating Cancer with Nutrition handy and refers to it often. "Beating Cancer with Nutrition is doable", he said. He has changed his diet, eats more natural foods, and drinks organic juices. J.B. has turned to Mind Body Medicine and believes he can heal himself. While his PSA is often a little high, he is still here, feels good and energetic. He goes to the gym 3x week, swims and walks regularly. J.B. is now 9 years beyond his diagnosis of a very poor prognostic cancer.

ENDNOTES

[1] https://www.who.int/nutrition/topics/vad/en/
[2] https://www.healthline.com/nutrition/foods/carrots#plant-compounds
[3] https://jech.bmj.com/content/56/11/813

KEY 2
UNDERSTAND THE SOLUTION

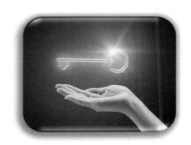

Chapter 2.1
Harnessing Your Innate Healing Forces
Nourishing the "Conductor" of Life

FROM NATURE'S PHARMACY: Pectin

When the nutritionists of the early 20th century found that a large part of plant food is indigestible fiber, they reasoned: "Since you cannot digest or absorb this stuff, then it must be useless, or even counterproductive." We now find that the value in fiber is its indigestible nature. Soluble fibers include pectin, and are extremely useful both in the human gut for health and in the food industry because pectin binds water and makes a gel like consistency in foods like jam and jelly. Pectin has been shown to reduce serum cholesterol while also feeding the friendly bacteria that help to produce vitamins (like biotin and K) and compete with the unfriendly bacteria and fungus that can turn our large intestines into a war zone. Nobel Prize winner Ilya Metchnikov in 1908 began the field of probiotics and prebiotics with his declaration "death begins in the colon." <u>70-80% of the body's immune system</u> resides in and around the colon. The health of our gut is crucial to our overall health. Pectin becomes a magical "broom" sweeping out the intestines of debris and pathogens before they can do any damage. With the generous amount of pectin in apples, maybe the old expression "an apple a day keeps the doctor away" has some merit. Pectin from citrus peelings has been processed to create "modified" citrus pectin, which has shown some activity against various forms of human cancer.

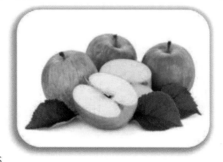

The story is told about Reverend Jones who was out in his garden one bright sunny spring morning. One of his parishioners walks by and says: "My, my Reverend Jones. Isn't it a beautiful garden that God has created for you?" To which Reverend Jones replies: "Yes, but you should have seen it before I got here." The point is, miracles are happening all around us and in us. And we must do our part to nourish those miracles, aka non-specific host defenses, homeostasis, dynamic equilibrium, autonomic functions. We cannot eat, drink, smoke, and move however we want and expect the "Conductor" to do its job. You must become a co-creator in the process of your health.

"What a piece of work is man…"
Shakespeare, Hamlet

The world's most complicated machine is the space shuttle, the taxi that takes payloads into space. With 2.5 million parts, this rocket blasts from zero to 17,000 MPH in 8 seconds. And this wonder of human accomplishment is child's play compared to your human body...the ultimate healing tool. Meet your body.

The world's most elegant and sophisticated symphony is going on inside of you right now. The average adult body has about 37 trillion cells, with 200 billion new cells produced daily to replace worn out tissue. In each of those cells, there are about 100,000 chemical reactions going on each second. Add another 100 trillion foreign microbes that inhabit your gut and other parts of your body in a hopefully, symbiotic relationship. Add in over 400 chemicals released by the brain and gut brain as part of your emotional reactions to your environment, with each of these chemicals having a "landing strip" on each of the above cells. Just try to imagine the interactions between the above cells and chemicals and you are beginning to understand the majesty of the human body.

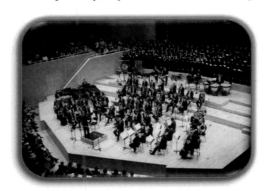

Brain

The 100 billion neurons in your brain each touch or have a synapse with 1000 other brain cells, yielding 100 trillion connections with, best guess, about a quadrillion bytes of data storage. That's 1 followed by 15 zeros. New research at Harvard [1] shows that brain plasticity probably increases memory storage capacity way beyond previous estimates. Research scientists spend a great deal of time and money trying to rule out the placebo effect, or the healing power of the brain. Some groups are moving aggressively to harness the healing power of the brain. More on that later in this book.

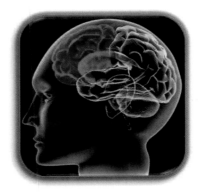

DNA

The 15 year $3 billion Human Genome Project (HGP), completed in 2003, was conducted by thousands of researchers around the world in 20 major universities. The 3 billion chemical units in the human DNA were data mined and thoroughly examined. The hope was in finding hard wiring in the DNA which could be fixed with brilliant gimmicks, such as that used to create genetically modified soy and corn.

Chimps and humans are 98.5% identical in DNA with mice being 97.5% identical in DNA to humans.[2] 99% of the human genome is considered "non-coding" or "junk".[3] Such arrogance. Just because we cannot decode it with current technology does not mean that 99% of the human DNA is junk. Remember, the DNA is like a spiral staircase in a lighthouse. It is 3 dimensional. The HGP stripped down the spiral staircase to a 2-dimensional ladder, then analyzed it. We have so much more to learn and appreciate about our "blueprints". Especially, the soft programming in the human DNA. Experts now speak of epigenetics,[4] or nutrigenomics, as ways of explaining how our environment interacts with the DNA to produce complex outcomes.

As an example of epigenetics, researchers took DNA samples from the prostate of men with slow growing (indolent) prostate cancer, then exposed these men to a lifestyle program of plant-based diet, exercise, and meditation. Three months later there were over <u>500 measurable changes in the DNA</u> [5] of the prostate after epigenetic lifestyle intervention. Google and Facebook have their algorithm, which is a complex math equation that determines who ends up high on the search engine. That algorithm is child's play compared to Nature's algorithm of life and health.

Gut

"With a little help from my friends..." sang the Beatles. In the petroleum age in which we live, oil refineries around the world take in crude black thick oil and render it into hundreds of different chemicals that can be used in modern society, including gasoline and plastics.

Child's play compared to the human gut. Humans take whole food and digest it down to molecules that can slide through the digestive wall, into the bloodstream, and be usable to the body. This is no small task.

The stomach produces acid that would eat a hole in your home carpet. But a healthy stomach can handle that. The intestines dump about a quart of digestive juices that take the necklace of your food, as polymers, and break it down to individual beads. Your digestive tract has the surface area of a tennis court. The large intestine contains most of the 100 million co-workers that scientists call the <u>microbiome</u>.[6] These microbes help to digest food, create vitamins (like biotin and K), generate extremely protective substances (like butyrate), and generally render exceptional service to you, the host, for the room and board that you provide them. Unless things get out of whack. Dysbiosis will be addressed later.

Breathing

Your lungs have the surface area of a tennis court and take in 11,000 liters of air daily to bring oxygen to the body cells. All this is done on automatic pilot while you sleep. Since oxygen is a powerful oxidizing agent, such as the effect on rusting nails and browning of cut apples, it is amazing that the lungs can usually protect themselves from the damaging effects of oxidation.

Bones

Your frame is built of 206 bones, with half of those bones in the hands and feet. Bones so hard that they mimic a helmet in the skull. Bones in the hands and feet are fluid and supple enough to play the violin, yet tough enough to break a brick if properly trained.

Heart

Your heart muscle is the size of your fist and beats 115,000 times per day to pump the 5 liters (roughly 1.5 gallons) of blood through 60,000 miles of blood vessels...thus bringing nutrients to your cells and carrying away waste products.

New Life

A female is born with 1-2 million immature eggs. Of those immature eggs, or follicles, only about 20 will mature per month in her fertility years, with one egg released during ovulation. A male will produce about 500 billion sperm cells in a lifetime with about 200 million in an ejaculation. If sperm fertilizes an egg inside the female, that one fertilized ovum will become several trillion cells in the next 9 months.

In Mother Nature's design the infant is delivered down mother's birth canal with mouth wide open to scoop up mother's microorganisms and begin to inoculate the sterile gut into with 100 trillion symbiotic organisms, kind of like baby's first "yogurt". Mother's body must make many compensations to provide fertile grounds for this new life within, including a stealth barrier around the fetus. 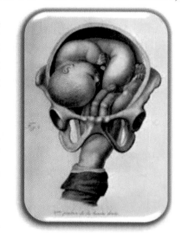 Normally, the immune system recognizes self from non self and destroys anything without your unique logo, or DNA. Yet the infant does not have mother's DNA, but a unique set of hybrid DNA from mother and father. Hence, the immune system must be put on hold to avoid destroying the fetus. Then mother must generate milk for the newly arrived infant. Human breast milk is a banquet of nutrients, immune factors, micro-vaccinations from pathogens that mother has been exposed to. All of this is beyond scientific explanation or replication.

Cancer

Cells divide, grow, mature, and die in a never-ending cycle of life and death throughout our lifetime. Bruce Ames, PhD at the University of California Berkeley has estimated that each human cell is exposed to roughly 10,000 <u>DNA hits per day</u>,[7] each a possible cancer-causing event. Imagine living in a category 5 hurricane while roof shingles were constantly being ripped from the roof, and you get to fix the problems during the ongoing hurricane. The human body says "no problem". That is why 60% of Americans will not end up in a cancer hospital. Yet, for the <u>40% of people in modern society who do develop cancer</u>,[8] take heart. There are many other mechanisms in place to help reverse cancer. Much more on that later.

If you are not at least a wee bit in awe of the above cursory explanation of the human body, then you are not paying attention.

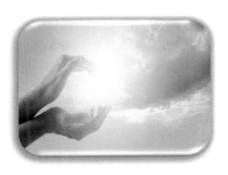

Modern medicine has the arrogance and ignorance to try to micromanage the above complex "soup" of life. We are not against emergency medicine providing life support and pain management. However, much of the $3.5 trillion medical industrial complex in America is driven by the sound bite: "manage symptoms with expensive and dangerous patented drugs." Ignore the Conductor.

But have no fear, the "Conductor" is here, aka the Life Force. The Conductor is what scientists refer to as "non-specific host defense mechanisms", or homeostasis, or dynamic equilibrium, or some vague polysyllabic phrase for: "we don't have a clue about how this works, but we can give it a name."

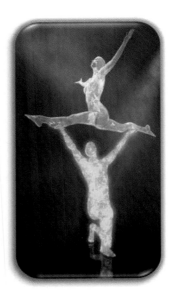

The Conductor is how people get well and stay well. If you provide the Conductor with all the necessary raw materials to do its job, and eliminate the interfering factors and forces that impair the Conductor, then health is the inevitable outcome. The Conductor will perform its job of healing and repairing your body...if you do your part.

For more information on how you can harness your own healing go to GettingHealthier.com

PATIENT PROFILE:

G.V. was originally diagnosed with breast cancer over 20 years ago. Then, at 58 G.V. was diagnosed with Stage 4 ovarian cancer. G.V. met with PQ after having been given a poor diagnosis by her Oncologist. "I was not in a good place at that time." Deciding she was going to take a different route, G.V. decided to change her lifestyle and diet. She had always been reasonably healthy but made many small changes. G.V. started seeing a Functional Medicine doctor. Dietary changes included eating mostly organic produce, eating grass fed beef (about 3oz daily), juicing, bone broth, <u>ImmunoPower</u> and other supplements. Other lifestyle changes include adding daily healing prayer, reducing stress, simplifying her life, and intermittent fasting, usually 16 hours a day. Breakfast is often coffee with cinnamon and MCT oil. Her day often starts with a workout at the gym. Many of the minor health issues, noticed by PQ, have since disappeared including a persistent cough. Today G.V. is a grandmother with 5 grandchildren who keep her busy. She has started a non-profit to teach children and teens the benefits of sustainable gardening. PQ helped her change her life for the better and was very encouraging from the outset. G.V. is now in remission and is feeling better than she has in 20 years. Her friends and family also say she looks healthier and younger.

ENDNOTES

[1] https://news.harvard.edu/gazette/story/2017/08/brain-flexibility-changes-the-way-we-remember-and-learn/

[2] https://www.newscientist.com/article/dn2352-just-2-5-of-dna-turns-mice-into-men/

[3] https://www.nytimes.com/2015/03/08/magazine/is-most-of-our-dna-garbage.html

[4] https://www.ncbi.nlm.nih.gov/pmc/articles/PMC1392256/

[5] http://www.pnas.org/content/105/24/8369

[6] https://www.ncbi.nlm.nih.gov/pmc/articles/PMC3709439/

[7] https://www.sciencedirect.com/science/article/pii/0027510789901966

[8] https://www.cancer.org/cancer/cancer-basics/lifetime-probability-of-developing-or-dying-from-cancer.html

KEY 2
UNDERSTAND THE SOLUTION

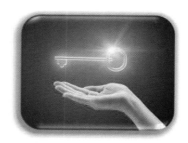

Chapter 2.2
Adaptive Forces of Nature (AFON)

"Nature to be commanded must be obeyed."
Francis Bacon, 1617, developer of the scientific method

FROM NATURE'S PHARMACY: Bananas

Few foods can rival the bonanza of nutrition found in a banana. Available nearly everywhere nearly any time of the year. Comes in it own wrapper, like nature's zip lock bag for a day trip. Grown in over 100 tropical countries throughout the world, the banana is 75% water and 25% solids, including a decent source of vitamin C, A, B-6 and magnesium; and a fantastic source of potassium...a mineral in which Americans are chronically deficient. Bananas have a low glycemic index (do not dramatically raise blood glucose) and provide a nice boost of mental and physical energy. A medium banana has 108 kcal, 1 gram of protein, negligible fat, and a rich source of pectin, a soluble fiber that helps with regularity and lowering cholesterol levels in the blood. Bananas are a favorite folk remedy for mild depression, premenstrual syndrome, hangovers, heartburn, obesity, and ulcers; use the inside of the peelings applied topically to accelerate healing of bug bites and warts. The FDA agrees with the ability of bananas to help lower blood pressure with its mighty potassium content. The pectin in a 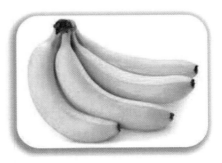 banana provides the "frosting on the cake" for many of my blender drinks. Throw in whatever fruits and vegetables into your high speed blender, then blend in ½ peeled banana for that smooth texture and keeping everything in solution. Peel bananas and freeze in a zip lock bag. Use ½ frozen banana to give your blender drinks a cold milkshake-like mouth feel. Great on hot summer days!

When Charles Darwin returned from his circumnavigation of the globe, his bright mind noticed the clear differences and similarities in plant and animal species around the world. His landmark book in 1859 ON THE ORIGIN OF SPECIES launched a maelstrom of debate. Some fundamentalists took great offence at any notion that humans could have evolved from apes. This debate was highlighted in the 1960 Hollywood film with Spencer Tracy "Inherit the Wind" where a courtroom watched the two sides offer their opinions.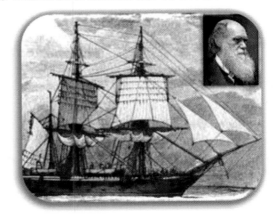

Personally, I see the Creator driving evolution, or adaptation. Random evolution creating a complex 37 trillion celled human from a single celled organism over the course of 4 billion years is as possible as a category 5 hurricane blowing through a Miami junkyard and creating a Boeing 747. Some Intelligence is at the helm in the ability of life to adapt to its region and stressors. Understanding these adaptive forces of nature is key to understanding how a human heals and what we need to maintain our ability to regulate and repair the incredible body human.

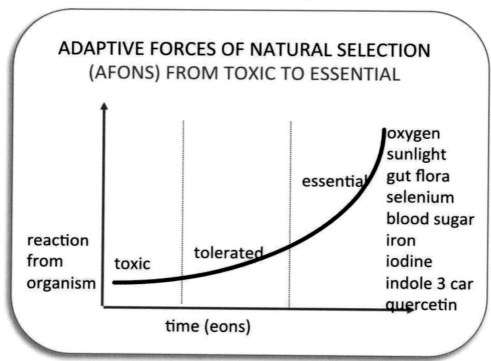

Black and White

Thick black hair and dark skin allow people to adapt to a sunny warm climate. Light hair and white skin allows people to adapt to a colder cloudy climate and still make some vitamin D from the meager sunlight offered. Eskimos have fat pads over their eyelids to allow them to adapt to subzero Arctic blasts of air. These are obvious examples of adapting to a region or climate. Let's move on.

Pollutants

The first and worst pollutant on the planet earth was oxygen. Biologists tell us that the primordial soup of life billions of years ago contained anaerobic (no oxygen) single cell organisms. One of those anaerobic cells mutated to develop chlorophyll, which then allowed that cell to capture energy from the sun in the process of photosynthesis. The byproduct or waste product of photosynthesis was oxygen, which destroyed all of the nearby cells in a rampage of free radicals. But eventually surrounding cells adapted to survive this harsh toxin of oxygen. Eventually, some organisms began using this oxygen in a far more efficient way of burning food as aerobic metabolism. Using oxygen, humans get "38 miles to the gallon" on food sources, while organisms that do not use oxygen only get 2 miles to the gallon. Higher forms of life were launched into the arena of earth. Humans and many other species are now heavily dependent on oxygen. Oxygen went from toxic to essential in a mere 4 billion years. More on that in the section on oxygen and cancer.

Here Comes the Sun

Sunlight is ionizing, mutagenic, carcinogenic radiation…and it is essential for human life. Humans adapted to move from tolerating sunlight to requiring sunlight. Sun on the skin generates vitamin D, which regulates at least 20% of the human genome, like a master conductor. Sun helps us to generate melatonin, which is crucial for sleep and regulating metabolism. People who work night shifts have higher levels of many health problems compared to people who get some sun during the day and sleep at night. Sun on the skin energizes the blood in the veins that are near the skin surface to create ultraviolet blood irradiation (UVBI), or a cleansing and

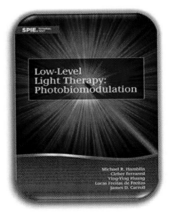

energizing of the immune system. <u>UVBI is used in many</u> forward thinking clinics around the world.[1]

Sunlight irrigates the retina of the eye to nourish and regenerate our health. The difference between a medicine and a poison is dosage. Sun exposure needs to be appropriate to the skin type. A suntan is good. A sunburn is bad. Humans adapted from tolerating to requiring sunlight.

Our energy generating stations within our cells, the mitochondria, have photoreceptors that make energy production more efficient in the presence of red light from the sun. Sunlight consists of the acronym ROY G. BIV of colors: red, orange, yellow, green, blue, indigo, violet. It is the red light that penetrates the skin and feeds our cells with renewed vitality. Put a flashlight on your hand and only the red light will penetrate through to the other side of your hand. AFONs explains the need for "appropriate" amounts of sunlight. We hide in our homes and offices, then cover our skin with clothing and makeup, then douse ourselves with sunscreen in those rare moments outside. You will be dazzled at the proven benefits of the 50,000 studies examining low level laser therapy (LLLT). More on sunlight in the section on Healthy Pleasures.

Paleolithic Diet

Our diet is composed of nutrients that our ancestors adapted to over the course of millennia. For 2 million years, humans ate wholesome food, mostly plant food, plenty of bacteria on the food, some animal food, and were exposed to frequent periods of fasting.

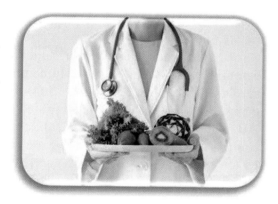

Many of the noxious substances in plant foods are naturally occurring pesticides, fungicides, and herbicides; which eventually became our modern field of chemoprevention through these phytochemicals. Modern medicine ignores these facts and assumes that you can take a patient who has deviated wildly from our native ancestral diet and load the patient with dangerous prescription drugs to mitigate the inevitable symptoms from this unhealthy diet.

Anthropologists tell us that the earliest human diet of 2 million years ago was fruit, eggs, and insects; which is what food could be obtained by our primitive ancestors. Well meaning health writers speak of the sugar in fruit as being the same problem as the refined sugar in ice cream, soda pop and desserts. All studies show the health benefits of whole fruit, which makes sense given the fact that we have adapted to need the phytochemicals, fiber, vitamins, and minerals in fruit. Indeed, all studies show that regular consumption of whole fruit lowers the risk for heart disease, obesity, diabetes, cancer, infections (like shingles), and more. Fruit is good for humans, which is what you would expect given the adaptive forces of nature.

Lectins

There has been considerable press and attention paid to lectins and the PLANT PARADOX, which states that these commonly present lectins in plant food pose health hazards for humans. Lectins are carbohydrate binding proteins found in most plant food, particularly whole grains and legumes. The proponents of these theories recommend avoiding these foods, and/or selecting white rice over whole grain rice, and/or buying their pills to bind up the lectin in the gut.

Meanwhile, all of the data on lectins shows that they have no adverse effects in humans. In fact, all of the data on the consumption of high lectin foods (whole grains and legumes) actually shows that these foods lower the risk for heart disease, diabetes, cancer, and more.[2] Which is what you would expect with AFON.

Indigenous People

Native Americans were primarily hunters who followed the enormous buffalo herds north in the summer and south in the winter. Things worked out reasonably well for 40,000 years until Europeans moved in and slaughtered the herds from 60 million buffalo down to the meager current 60,000. Take those people who adapted to live on grass fed meat, then provided with federal government compensation of food stamp program consisting of white flour, white sugar, instant mashed potatoes, and other non-foods and you have the makings for a health catastrophe...which is exactly what happened to these once proud hunters. Obesity, diabetes, alcoholism, and more have increased exponentially by ignoring the AFON of Native Americans.

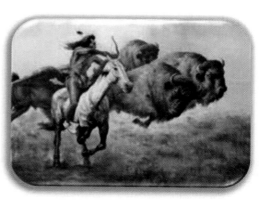

Same thing happened to the Aborigines of Australia. Professor of nutrition Kerrin O'Dea took 10 obese diabetic Aborigines, returned them to <u>their native diet</u>, and presto, their health returned to normal.[3] Same thing happened to Eskimos, or Native Americans from the Arctic region. 40,000 years of living off high fat seafood, then switched to the junk carb diet of Americans and health problems galore have surfaced. African Americans have descended from native groups in Africa that were exposed to frequent famines. Give those people unlimited access to junk carbohydrate foods, then take away the tropical sunshine that gave them vitamin D and you have the makings of another health catastrophe, which is exactly what is happening to African Americans: much higher incidence of obesity, diabetes, heart disease, cancer, and more.

Animal Foods

Explorers and scientists have never found a strict vegan group anywhere in the world. There are plenty of people who choose veganism for spiritual or religious reasons, which is fine. But throughout history, people who added some animal food (meat, eggs, dairy) to their diet were usually healthier, due to the carnivore nutrients of zinc, iron, B-12, carnitine, EPA, cartilage, and more.

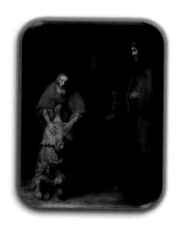

Some groups ate lots of meat. Most ate little, such as the Biblical reference (Luke 15:29) to the killing of the fatted calf in the return of the prodigal son. Eating meat was a celebration, not a common event. The herd animals were an important part of the tribe, providing dairy (milk, butter, cheese, yogurt). The male animals were for breeding and protecting the herd. The female animals were for breeding and dairy. Killing the animal means no more of the above.

Take that same model of AFON for the cows, which are ruminants adapted to a grass diet, and feed them GMO corn, plus plenty of antibiotics and hormones to get them fatter quicker, then lock their heads in a vice so they cannot roam around, then you have very sick animals from acidosis. They need antibiotics just to stay alive for their brief life. Take the meat from those animals and you have a very different nutritional profile compared to free range animals.

When the farmer slaughtered an animal, the only thing that was wasted was the squeal. Every part was eaten. Sausage was the process of taking less tasty meats that are very nutritious (liver, heart, kidney, etc.) and grinding it up, then add medicinal spices (black pepper, cardamom, all spice, cilantro, anything from the herb garden). Sausage used to be a nourishing food. Not anymore. You now have the high fat part of the meat, which is where many of the toxins accumulate from the animal's unhealthy environment, and sugar.

Dairy

The most perfect food on earth for a newborn mammal is mother's milk. Whole fresh unprocessed milk contains a rich mixture of immunoglobulins for immunity and maturation of the gut lining, which get destroyed by the pasteurization process. It is illegal to sell non-pasteurized milk in many states. Fresh milk also contains the perfect fats for making a cell membrane that properly conducts electricity, until you force those fats through a tiny aperture, aka homogenized milk. Now those once invaluable fats are mere shards of their original chemical structure. If you ordered a pane of glass to replace your broken window in your home and the delivery person brought you a box of shattered glass, would you be able to repair the window?

Ikaria is an island off the coast of Greece where people <u>regularly live to 90</u>.[4] These people eat a Mediterranean diet of vegetables, greens, fruits, whole grains (pasta), olive oil, legumes and small amounts of meat, fish, and dairy. Their dairy is from goat's milk, which provides a different nutrient profile than commercial cow's milk. Take that same unhealthy agri-business cow mentioned above and the dairy from that animal may not be good for humans. The grass fed goats for the Ikarians are very nourishing, including the conjugated linoleic acid that has anti-cancer, anti-heart disease merit.

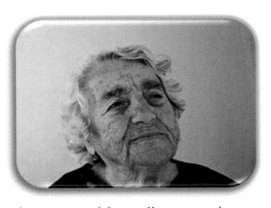

While whole milk consumption in men definitely increases the risk of prostate cancer, the data on other forms of dairy show a slight decrease in cancer risk with small amounts of cheese, yogurt, and butter. Meanwhile, saturated fats from meat and dairy are clear risk factors for the autoimmune disease multiple sclerosis.[5] Your author has found that yogurt is often the only remedy for diarrhea induced by pelvic radiation (between the hips for prostate or colon cancer) and other digestive disturbances. AFON would predict that small amounts of dairy products from healthy grass fed animals would be healthy for most humans.

Catching Fire

In our 2 million years of roaming the earth, humans discovered fire about a million years ago. Fire allowed people to stay warm, light the night, scare off predators, and cook their food. Cooked food, like oatmeal, allows us to extract 60% more calories from the food. Cooked buffalo allowed our ancestors to consume more calories and protein and develop a larger brain with smaller gut. Ruminants are animals that have a multi-chambered stomach and are vegans. Up to one third the weight of a ruminant, such as a goat, is gut for digesting the indigestible. Plant cells are coated in

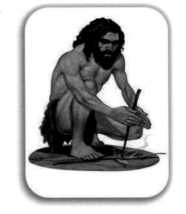

cellulose which is indigestible to most animals. Ruminants rely on trillions of microbes in their gut in a symbiotic relationship to make the enzyme, cellulase, to digest plant cells. In cooking food, we burst open the plant cell to release the contents for nourishment. According to <u>Harvard scientist Richard Wrangham, PhD</u>, the discovery of cooking food allowed humans to rise above the rest of the animal kingdom with a big brain and smaller gut.[6] CATCHING FIRE: HOW COOKING MADE US HUMAN, may disturb the raw food advocates, but is scientifically valid.

Most fruits and some vegetables are best eaten raw. Cooking meat and fish eliminates the parasites while making the food easier to chew and digest. Even the most primitive societies on earth cook their food. When you understand AFONs, this all makes sense.

Fasting

Regular meals are a very recent phenomenon in human existence. For 2 million years our ancestors spent much of their waking hours searching for food. Hunger was a common state. Because of this, natural adaptation created rejuvenating mechanisms that work best within us when we fast for a day or so. The long lived Ikarians of Greece consider regular fasting an important part of their lifestyle, where 1/3 of these people live past 90.

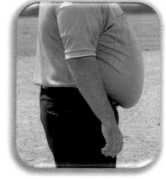

Think about it. A million years ago, one of your ancestors was really hungry. Nature created AFON that make that person smarter, younger, and faster to find some food...or die. Autophagy is the state of the body scrapping marginal cells to create younger and more vibrant cells...in order to find some food. Modern humans eat too much, too often, and the wrong foods. It is the "too often" that is killing us as much as too much and the wrong foods.

Due to excessive eating, insulin and blood glucose are constantly pounding on the cell membrane, which creates insulin resistance. Stop eating. Just for a day. Watch how your body regenerates itself. I was one of the 60 million Americans with prediabetic symptoms of fasting blood glucose in the 100 mg/dl range. The only therapy that switched me into extremely healthy fasting blood glucose was fasting. One day a week consume nothing but water. Have a greater gap between your last meal at night and first meal in the morning, or "break fast". Watch your health flourish.

Omnivorous Plant Based Diet
"Now be fruitful and multiply and repopulate the earth."
Genesis 9:7

Humans are built for diaspora, or the dispersion of people from their homeland, like dandelion seeds into the wind. Tracking the exploration of the earth by early humans has been a breathtaking study. Thor Heyerdahl built and sailed a handmade raft 5000 miles from South America to Polynesia in 1947. There have been many similar expeditions since proving how early humans colonized the earth via the conveyer of the oceans. And do you know what these people ate as they explored the world? Whatever they could find.

There have been quite a few self-appointed experts on nutrition recently who have advocated various extreme diets: all vegan, all raw, no grains or legumes, high fat and protein, low fat and little protein, no fruit, no lectins (found in all plant food), eat white rice instead of brown rice, etc. Humans are the ultimate in "flex fuel" creatures. While a flex fuel 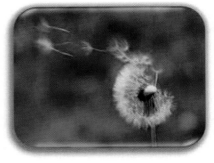 car can run on gasoline or ethanol (alcohol from corn), humans can run on almost anything edible. Survival experts who teach soldiers how to survive in the wild essentially reduce their final lecture to: "eat whatever doesn't eat you first."

From scorching desserts of 120 F (49 C) and sauna bath jungles to the Siberian town where average winter temperatures can reach minus 58F (-50C). Humans live there. Only because we can eat almost anything.

Doesn't mean that we should eat almost anything. That is another discussion. However, a healthy human gut has a remarkable capacity to digest nearly any real food. Note the qualifying statement of "a healthy human gut…real food."

Fiber is indigestible plant matter. You cannot digest or absorb fiber, and because of that fiber is essential because fiber (prebiotic) feeds the 100 trillion microbes in the gut that play a powerful role in our health. The microbiome is ground zero for a healthy human gut and is discussed in detail in another chapter. AFON says that humans had to adapt to a wide variety of food and needed the assistance from commensal organisms in the gut in order to colonize the planet earth. Get your gut healthy and adverse reactions to real food are rare.

Fermented Foods

For 2 million years our ancestors spent much of their waking hours searching for food. This food was not clean. It was full of bacteria. Once these people found some plant or animal food, keeping the extra food was a challenge. Drying and salting the meat slowed down spoilage. But plant food could be fermented using naturally available bacteria to 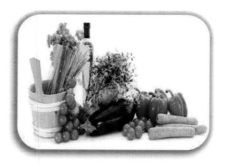 generate an acidic environment around the food to discourage spoilage. Sauerkraut, yogurt, kimchi, pickles and other foods are examples of commonly available fermented foods. From these foods our ancestors found nourishment as acids that aid in digestion and trillions of microorganisms to colonize the gut and compete with pathogenic organisms. Humic and fulvic acids are by-products of bacterial fermentation in the soil and fermented foods and provide extraordinary ways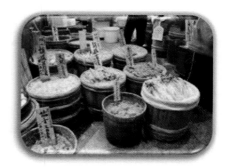

of enhancing agricultural production in the land and health in your body. <u>Fermented foods</u> are high in humic and fulvic acid, which are potent stimulators of human health.[7] Hence, fermented foods and eating bacteria are almost essential for human health via the AFONs principle.

In her book GUT AND PSYCHOLOGY SYNDROME, neurologist and mother of an autistic son, Natasha Campbell-McBride, MD found that fermented foods could help restore health to a diseased gut and helped to heal her autistic son. Sandor Katz has compiled a brilliant review of the whole subject of fermenting almost any food in THE ART OF FERMENTATION. There is compelling evidence that <u>extreme hygiene during childhood</u> is a risk factor for childhood allergies and autoimmune diseases.[8] There is such a thing as being too clean. AFON explains this conundrum nicely.

Sleep

Sleep is an essential ingredient for human health. Most adults in America stagger around with chronic sleep deprivation, which generates cortisol, the stress hormone. The inhumane interrogation of prisoners of war often involves sleep deprivation, which breaks down the body, mind, and spirit. Night shifts increase the risk for obesity, injuries, and numerous health problems.[9] We are built to require 8 hours of sleep at night. Ignore that rule and you will suffer many health consequences. AFON explains this.

Blood Donors Wanted

Iron is an essential mineral in human nutrition and one of the more common minerals that is deficient in the human diet. When iron in the body is bound to protein carriers, such as hemoglobin, it performs essential tasks. When iron is unbound, often due to acidosis, iron becomes a wrecking ball in the human body.

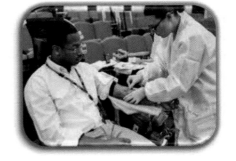

Iron is a free radical generator, just like watching a nail rust outside, iron can "rust" in your body and generate free radicals, which can lead to disease and premature aging. Creatures with hemoglobin are heavily dependent on iron for life, which also can become an assassin within.

Humans are built to bleed. Our ancestors were regularly exposed to bleeding from injuries, war, and animal attacks. Hence, humans built a "factory" in our bone marrow for constantly making red blood cells. If we don't bleed, especially adult men, then our blood becomes packed and thick in viscosity. Regular (at least yearly) donation of blood <u>lowers cardiovascular risk factors</u> by lowering cholesterol and iron content.[10] Donating blood <u>lowers the risk</u> for cancer.[11] Blood donation even lowers risk factors for inflammation (CRP) and <u>raises antioxidant capacity</u>.[12]

It all makes sense. Humans are built to bleed. Our ancestors did so inadvertently. Because of AFONs, we can reap the health benefits of blood donation, while also enjoying the psychological <u>benefits of altruism and benevolence</u>.[13]

Bottom Line

Over the course of eons, humans have adapted to require certain factors to keep our body healthy. Unadulterated, unprocessed food, primarily plant based; sunlight, sleep, companionship, low stress, activity, minimal toxins, etc. Modern humans have violated most of the above adaptive needs for humans, then we wonder why 42% of modern humans will get cancer in their lifetime and <u>88% of Americans</u> [14] have some metabolic disease.

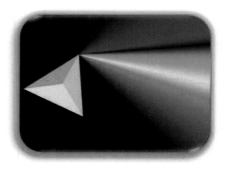

Adaptive forces of nature provide the missing answers in healthcare. Full spectrum light includes all the colors. Full spectrum healing includes all the modalities mentioned in this book. You can use your body the way it was designed by the Creator, or ignore these rules of nature and suffer the consequences.

For more information about the adaptive forces of nature go to <u>GettingHealthier.com</u>

PATIENT PROFILE

J.G. was initially diagnosed with colon cancer in 2015. He had a phone consultation with PQ on May 25, 2018 during the time he was doing chemotherapy. J.G. started exercising and improved his eating habits, with a more plant-based diet. He also increased his supplement intake and still takes various supplements. Today J.G. is in remission. He feels really good.

ENDNOTES

[1] https://www.ncbi.nlm.nih.gov/pmc/articles/PMC4783265/
[2] https://www.sciencedirect.com/science/article/pii/S0733521014000228
[3] https://www.ncbi.nlm.nih.gov/pubmed/6373464
[4] https://www.bluezones.com/exploration/ikaria-greece/
[5] https://www.ncbi.nlm.nih.gov/pmc/articles/PMC6132382/
[6] https://www.amazon.com/Catching-Fire-Cooking-Made-Human-ebook/dp/B0097D71MQ/ref=sr_1_1?keywords=richard+wrangham+book+on+catching+fire&qid=1565123076&s=gateway&sr=8-1
[7] http://www.integratedhealthblog.com/tag/fermented-foods/
[8] https://onlinelibrary.wiley.com/doi/full/10.1111/j.1365-2567.2004.01925.x
[9] https://onlinelibrary.wiley.com/doi/abs/10.1002/rnj.107
[10] https://www.ncbi.nlm.nih.gov/pmc/articles/PMC3663474/
[11] https://academic.oup.com/jnci/article/100/8/572/927859
[12] https://www.degruyter.com/view/j/jbcpp.2016.27.issue-6/jbcpp-2015-0111/jbcpp-2015-0111.xml
[13] https://www.mentalhealth.org.uk/publications/doing-good-altruism-and-wellbeing-age-austerity
[14] https://www.sciencedaily.com/releases/2018/11/181128115045.htm

KEY 3
GENETICS

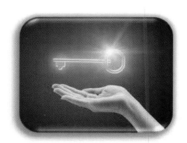

Chapter 3
Epigenetics
Making the Most of the Cards
You Were Dealt

"Each patient carries his own doctor inside him." Albert Schweitzer, MD, Nobel laureate 1940

FROM NATURE'S PHARMACY: Lutein

Macular degeneration is a blindness that affects almost 2 million Americans, mostly over age 65. There is a growing body of data showing that lutein and its cousin carotenoid zeaxanthin may be able to prevent or delay the onset of macular degeneration. Lutein is an orange colored substance found mostly in green vegetables and used by plants as part of photosynthesis. In the human eye, lutein is used as a "buffer" or antioxidant to reduce the damage from blue light on the "screen" of the eye, the retina. Best sources of lutein include leafy greens (like spinach, kale, collards), broccoli, zucchini, peas, corn, Brussels sprouts. Most Americans do not get enough lutein.

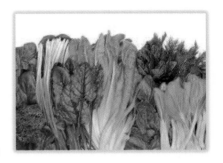

"Like Begets Like."

Since the dawn of time, humans were well aware of the similarities between parents and children. Farmers know that bringing a healthy bull into the stockyard can enhance the vitality of the herd. Osama bin Laden was the 17th of 52 children born from his father. One of the "fruits" of a conqueror was the ability to breed with many women, allegedly producing more children like the victorious father. Sobhuza was an African leader in Swaziland who had 70 wives and 210 children over his 80 year reign of power. Although Genghis Khan died 750 years ago, one geneticist claims that 16 million men in China bear Khan's unique Y chromosome. Khan was quite a lover and conqueror.

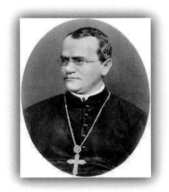

Casual observance led the late 19th century Austrian monk Gregor Mendel to carefully experiment with pea plants to note their units of inheritance, thus founding the modern science of genetics. In 1953 James Watson and Francis Crick earned the Nobel Prize for their explanation of the double helix molecule of DNA, looking like a spiral staircase. In 2003 the $5 billion Human Genome Project wrapped up a 15-year massive research project conducted in 20 universities around the world. It was hoped that the results of this massive research project would reveal the inner workings of our DNA or blueprint, thus allowing scientists to create targeted drugs to tweak specific defects in our DNA. If science can genetically modify corn and soy, then why can't we modify the human

DNA for the better? The results of this project were more and less than anyone could have expected.

Experts still cannot agree on how many protein coding genes are in the human DNA, with estimates ranging between 20,000 and 100,000. According to the prevailing opinion, more than 90% of human DNA is "junk" or non-coding material. Problem is that the experts are looking at this three-dimensional structure of a spiral staircase human DNA by laying it flat, like a ladder, thus losing its stereochemistry and much of the information that is no doubt hiding in the intact three-dimensional structure. According to this massive research project, humans share 97.5% identical DNA with mice. If you find those results disappointing, then join the club.

In 2013, Hollywood star Angelina Jolie underwent a preventive bilateral mastectomy because her mother died of cancer at age 56 and Angelina tested positive for the BRCA1 gene. Current opinion among conservative experts is that 5-10% of cancer is genetically driven, the rest is lifestyle induced.

Make no mistake. Genetics are a powerful force. Enter the emerging science of epigenetics.[1] "Epi" means above. Our genes can be adjusted, molded, modified by lifestyle. Most people will never play in the NFL due to their genes (DNA), but most people do not have to die from the same conditions as their ancestors (epigenetics). Most diseases are a collision of genes with lifestyle. About 14% of the western population test positive for APOE4, which increases the risk for Alzheimer's disease. Doesn't mean you are going to get Alzheimer's, it just means that lifestyle factors now become the "blasting caps" for the dynamite of this genetic factor. Dale Bredesen, MD [2] at UCLA has done pioneering work in reversing Alzheimer's disease through lifestyle, detoxification, hormone balancing and other modifiable parameters in the human body. You need both the APOE4 gene and unhealthy lifestyle to get Alzheimer's.

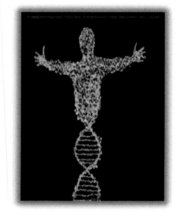

The HLA-DRB1 gene increases the risk for multiple sclerosis, but you need to add lifestyle risks of low vitamin D, etc in order to develop MS. I am of Irish descent, with fair skin. In Ireland, my ancestors used this fair skin advantage to generate more vitamin D from less sun. Take that same fair skin and bring it to the farm fields of Illinois where I worked outside in the summer sun after nine months in the classroom, then the beaches of southern California where I swim and bike and you have the blasting caps and dynamite for skin cancer. And I have dealt with basal and squamous cell cancers. Doesn't mean that I was doomed to skin cancer from birth. Means that I needed to add the environmental insult of many sunburns to make skin cancer.

Same with most other cancers. You may have inherited a genetic vulnerability to cancer, but you can do something about it through lifestyle changes as outlined in this book. Dr. Dean Ornish is a cardiologist who wearied of doing second and third bypass surgeries on his patients and asked the obvious question: "Can we prevent or reverse heart disease through lifestyle?" By 1998, Dr. Ornish had compiled irrefutable

CAN LIFESTYLE IMPROVE THE REPAIR OF DEFECTIVE DNA (CANCER)?

Study design: 30 men with indolent prostate cancer (PSA 4.8) were assessed for gene expression profiles from prostate cancer needle biopsy at DX and 3 months after beginning intervention lifestyle program.
Results: Micro arrays detected 48 up regulated and 453 down regulated transcripts after intervention. Side benefits included: inc.mental health, dec. BMI, BP, LDL, chol*, triglyc, CRP, waist line (8 cm)

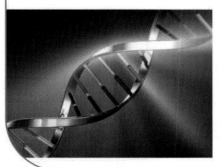

Intervention:
Diet (plant based, whole food, low fat 11% kcal)
Exercise (3.6 hr/wk)
Stress management (4.5 hr/wk)

CONCLUSIONS: This pilot study is the first to show genetic changes in cancer patients based solely on lifestyle intervention.
Ornish, et al., PNAS, 105, 24, June 17, 2008

evidence [3] that heart disease can be reversed through a low fat vegan diet combined with meditation and exercise. Dr. Ornish then asked the same question for prostate cancer, the most common cancer in American men: "Can lifestyle slow or reverse prostate cancer?" The answer is yes. By using the same lifestyle intervention of a low fat vegan diet coupled with meditation and exercise, the 30 participants in this 3 month intervention trial experienced an average of 500 genetic changes, which were all moving in the direction of reversing indolent prostate cancer. [4]

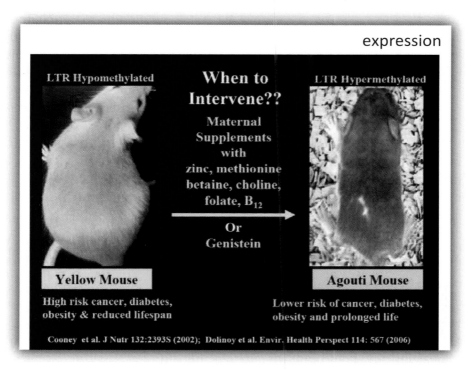

expression

When to Intervene??

Maternal Supplements with zinc, methionine betaine, choline, folate, B_{12}

Or Genistein

LTR Hypomethylated

LTR Hypermethylated

Yellow Mouse

High risk cancer, diabetes, obesity & reduced lifespan

Agouti Mouse

Lower risk of cancer, diabetes, obesity and prolonged life

Cooney et al. J Nutr 132:2393S (2002); Dolinoy et al. Envir. Health Perspect 114: 567 (2006)

All mammals have an agouti gene. A strain of mice have been specially bred to have an unmethylated agouti gene, which makes them prone toward obesity, diabetes, and cancer; thus commonly used in research. In 2004, researchers at Duke University fed high doses of methylation nutrients [5] (methionine, choline, folic acid, B12, B6) to pregnant Agouti mice and were able to change the color of fur and predisposition to obesity and diabetes in the offspring. One study found that early nutrition has a major <u>epigenetic influence on the newborn</u> [6] through changes in the microbiome in the gut.

Genes are like switches on the wall. You turn them on and off with various lifestyle issues. We have a gene that turns on another gene that makes fingers while we are in utero. Then another gene turns off that gene which says "make fingers" once we reach the quota of 10 fingers. In <u>Minerals for the Genetic Code</u>,[7] the author shows how minerals in our diet turn on and off various genes in our DNA, making mineral deficiencies an underlying cause for some cancers. <u>Professor Bruce Ames of UC Berkeley asserts</u> [8] that low intake of micronutrients (e.g. folate, vitamin C, vitamin A) create fragile DNA which eventually leads to cancer and premature aging. There is an abundance of data showing that <u>many dietary factors</u> [9] (e.g. vitamin D, folate, resveratrol, green tea EGCG) can affect genetic expression.

Nutrigenomics and epigenetics allow us the "get out of jail free" card to avoid the health pitfalls of our ancestors. All of this information should be good news to cancer patients and family members. You are not a prisoner of your genes. Epigenetics means "above your genes". Lifestyle plays a prominent role in your genetic expression of diseases. You can have a huge influence on turning on or off the various genes that regulate disease. You can beat cancer by upregulating your body's own natural healing forces. The trump card in disease is you.

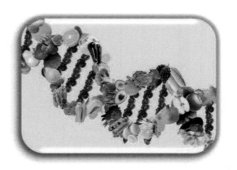

For more information about genetics and making the most of the cards you are dealt, go to <u>GettingHealthier.com.</u>

PATIENT PROFILE

MAC was initially diagnosed with 2B breast cancer in 2009. PQ had a phone consultation with MAC in May 2015 at a time when she was very weak. Though she is not feeling 100% and experiences nausea and dizziness due to her medication, she is leading a more normal life. She is currently taking many supplements including selenium, 8000 IU Vitamin D, maitake mushroom, NAC, olive leaf extract, alpha lipoic acid, CO10 and a pea-based protein drink daily. She believes her daily juicing contributed significantly to her recovery. She is currently in remission.

ENDNOTES

[1] https://www.scirp.org/Journal/PaperInformation.aspx?PaperID=87660

[2] https://www.amazon.com/End-Alzheimers-Program-Prevent-Cognitive/dp/0735216207/ref=sr_1_1?crid=2AVT192L78I27&keywords=dale+bredesen%27s+book+the+end+of+alzheimer%27s&qid=1555360652&s=gateway&sprefix=dale+bredesen%2Caps%2C199&sr=8-1

[3] https://jamanetwork.com/journals/jama/article-abstract/188274

[4] https://www.pnas.org/content/105/24/8369.short

[5] https://wolfweb.unr.edu/homepage/zehd/Waterland&Jirtle2004.pdf

[6] https://www.cambridge.org/core/journals/nutrition-research-reviews/article/epigenetic-mechanisms-elicited-by-nutrition-in-early-life/5B88564391393FB040316DDDBEC2F73C

[7] https://www.amazon.com/dp/B00SM1MCPU/ref=dp-kindle-redirect?_encoding=UTF8&btkr=1

[8] https://www.pnas.org/content/103/47/17589?eaf=

[9] https://bpspubs.onlinelibrary.wiley.com/doi/pdf/10.1111/j.1476-5381.2012.02002.x

KEY 4
ATTITUDE/THE MIND

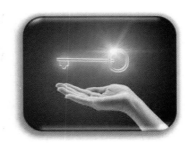

Chapter 4
Your Mind: The Ultimate Healing Force

"A cheerful heart is good medicine, but a crushed spirit dries up the bones." Proverbs 17:22

"Every cell in your body is eavesdropping on your thoughts."
Deepak Chopra, MD

FROM NATURE'S PHARMACY: Turmeric

    For over 4000 years, Indian people have used curry to season their food. Indian Ayurvedic medicine has used curry as a favorite medicine. Curry is a blend of herbs, like the recipe for chocolate chip cookies...everyone has their own version. Turmeric, red pepper, black pepper, and cumin are common ingredients in curry spice. Turmeric is the bright yellow herb also found in mustard. Turmeric is rich in curcumin, which has active ingredients called curcuminoids. These yellow substances have a list of biological activity that would make any drug company president drool with envy: anti-cancer, anti-arthritic, liver protective, anti-inflammatory, anti-viral, slows Alzheimer's, and treats malaria. Researchers then found that turmeric is poorly absorbed...unless you add black pepper, which dramatically enhances the absorption of turmeric. Note the above 4000-year old recipe for curry 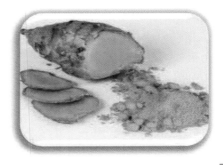 mixes turmeric and black pepper. Start using curry with turmeric in many of your foods. You are practicing herbal medicine without a license.

For thousands of years mystics, healers, and philosophers have noticed the powerful link between our thoughts and our physical health. According to the US Center for Disease Control, 90% [1] of our $3.5 trillion dollar medical dilemma is produced by stress and people with mental ailments. Big Pharma spends billions of dollars each year in research trying to eliminate the "placebo effect", which basically says that the therapy works because you believe it works. At least 30% of all modern medicine, from drugs through surgery, works because of the placebo effect. Rather than trying to eliminate the placebo effect, let's harness it for your own healing. Many talented scientists and clinicians are measuring and implementing the healing power of the mind, in fields called psychoneuroimmunology, mind/body medicine, mindfulness, etc.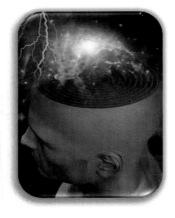

The Human Mind

"Our deepest fear is not that we are inadequate. Our deepest fear is that we are powerful beyond measure."
Marianne Williamson

"What a piece of work…" wrote Shakespeare about the human body. And the mind is the penultimate creation of the human body. The human brain consists of around 100 billion nerve cells, each of which has connections with another 1000 other nerve cells, making about 100 trillion connections or synapses that are, allegedly, responsible for our memory and brain function. But any honest neurosurgeon will admit the limitations of our understanding or ability to repair the human brain.

The brain is a <u>3 pound organ</u>,[2] which consists of 75% water and the remaining tissue is 60% fat. The blood vessels in the human brain, if stretched end to end, would be over 100,000 miles long. As dazzling as these statistics are, it doesn't begin to explain how a person can memorize any exquisite piano concerto. Or how creativity works in geniuses. Or how clairvoyance, dreams predicting the future, or non-verbal communication works. Or how a seasoned meditator can defy the laws of medicine and put themselves into suspended animation. Once we realize that we are more than our 3 pound brain, we begin to embrace the inescapable conclusion of the human mind, which is far more encompassing than just the brain.

How Psychological Stress Affects the Body

Hans Selye, MD (1907-1982) was a Canadian physician and researcher who first documented the physical effects of psychological stress. His career included publishing 1700 research articles and 7 popular books and was nominated for the Nobel Prize in 1949. In the 1940s Selye took rats and tied them to a table. No pain, just took away their freedom for 24 hours. He then sacrificed and autopsied these animals with the striking results that they had the beginnings of ulcers (atrophy of the gastric mucosa), beginnings of heart disease (elevated cholesterol), swelling of the adrenal cortex (adrenal burnout), beginnings of cancer and premature aging (atrophy of the thymus gland).

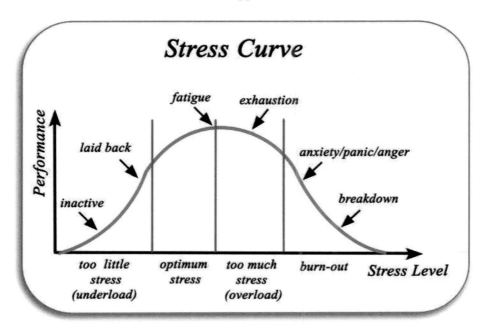

Selye became an armchair philosopher in his later years with popular books, including The Stress of Life and Stress without Distress. He explained that humans are built to withstand brief and rare moments of stress. Our ancestors were confronted by the tiger. We must "fight or flight". Our bodies are built to engage in that brief pivotal encounter with danger. We react perfectly. Our blood pressure increases. Our heart races. Our blood thickens to allow for the inevitable need to clot our blood once the tiger takes a bite out of us. Our bowels and bladder empty. If we survive this brief encounter, then no harm done.

The problem is that modern humans are exposed to nearly endless stress. Not enough money, kids are giving us trouble, boss at work is a pain, marriage is on the rocks, crowded commute to work, etc. The constant flow of cortisol, the stress hormone, is like continuously whipping a race horse. Eventually, the horse tires and falls down. There are many solutions to this issue of stress that are discussed throughout this book, starting with changing your attitude and/or venue and meditating.

Dr. Selye offered some valuable advice for us to make stress a good thing in our lives (eustress).

✓ Lean on a higher power. Selye found that people who attempt to micro-manage their life end up burned out.

✓ Know your personal speed in life. There are "race horses" who are stressed when they stop their 16 hour work day. There are "turtles" who need far more rest, slower pace, and more time alone. Know your individual tempo needs and work accordingly.

STRESS RESPONSE SYSTEM

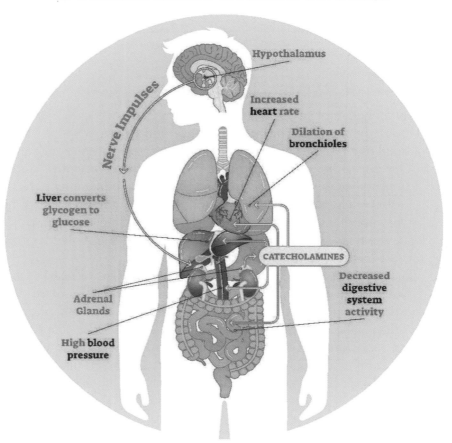

✓ Altruistic egotism.   Help others with the ultimate end goal of the process,   eventually   helping yourself.
✓ Stress is like the tension on a violin string. Just enough tension and the string brings sweet music. Not enough tension and there is no music. Too much tension and the string breaks.

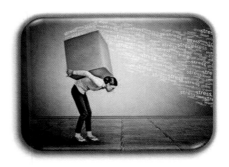

For many cancer patients, stress was the final breaking point. We can succumb to the pressures of life, or create a new low stress bubble for ourselves. Many a cancer patient has found relief and even healing when they assume a new attitude on life.

Spooky Science

"Physics is the only real science. The rest are just stamp collecting."
Ernest Rutherford, PhD (1871-1937)
Nobel Prize winning physicist and father of the modern nuclear age

Dr. Rutherford's brilliance might be humbled by the modern field of quantum mechanics, which states that 99.9999% of all matter is space, and the remaining fragment that claims to be solid matter, actually fluctuates between particle and wave and has been called "frozen light". What Einstein once called "spooky" is now the new physics, where the lines between physics and spirituality and healing blur. Russell Targ, PhD, Stanford physicist and consultant with the CIA and Department of Defense for decades, has written a fantastic book <u>THE REALITY OF ESP</u>:[3] A PHYSICIST'S PROOF OF PSYCHIC ABILITIES, in which he explains how most physicists today embrace the notion of non-local consciousness…some vague connection throughout the universe.

There is an energy cloud that exists throughout space and time. And we can tap into this energy cloud through our mind. Dr. Targ pioneered work on remote viewing, where trained and gifted psychics could "see" with their mind's eye situations thousands of miles away.

They solved murders. They saw into high security military operations of other countries. Distance made no difference. Nor did placing the psychic in a lead shielded cage. We are all connected in an elegant web of energy. We simply need to learn how to focus this unlimited energy.

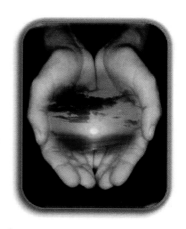

Since 1967, the <u>University of Virginia</u> [4] School of Medicine has conducted studies on this vague notion of consciousness through their Department of Perceptual Studies. For a half century, many very bright scientists have gathered conclusive evidence that:

"consciousness may indeed survive bodily death and that mind and brain appear to be distinct and separable."

The <u>Heart Math Institute</u> [5] began by collecting data on the link between stress and heart disease, but have expanded well beyond that solid principle: "into balanced alignment with their heart's intuitive guidance". Edgar Mitchell, PhD was considered the unflappable astronaut when he became one of only 12 people to set foot on the moon in 1971. His return trip home brought an epiphany that made him feel connected to all. Dr. Mitchell co-founded the <u>Institute of Noetic Sciences</u> [6] and spent his remaining years using his bright mind to study physics, consciousness, and unexplained phenomena.

In the science fiction classic movie from the 1950s, <u>Forbidden Planet</u>, astronauts find a stranded scientist with a device that has unlimited capacity to create, if the user can connect his/her mind to the device. What if we have the capacity to connect to a vast unlimited Source of power to change our world, individually and collectively?

What does all this ethereal nonsense have to do with your healing? A lot. Maybe the trump card that will get you well. Kelly Turner, PhD wrote a brilliant book, <u>RADICAL REMISSIONS</u>, [7] in which she interviewed 70 cancer patients from around the world who experienced a complete remission from their documented stage 4 cancer without any conventional treatment. Dr. Turner found that these people had 9 common strategies that help beat their cancer, of which 2 were nutrition (plant-based diet, herbals) and the remaining 7 strategies were psycho-spiritual. They changed their way of thinking. No oncologist can explain this, and few will even listen to it.

"These works you can do and more." John 13:12

Or we could talk about Dr. Joe Dispenza, the young chiropractor who had his spine shattered in a biking accident. Joe was told by his physician that he would never walk again. Joe went within for his healing. He spent 2 hours twice daily meditating to find the "space within the space (peace)" for 12 weeks, and was then walking and lifting weights. His books have been inspirational for many patients and healers.

Or we could trot out in front of the jury a book by Lissa Rankin, MD <u>MIND OVER MEDICINE</u>[8] in which this physician compiles the overwhelming evidence that our mind can be a powerful tool in the healing process. Decades of research and clinical insight from healers like Bruce

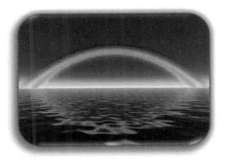

Lipton, PhD and Deepak Chopra, MD have shown the forgotten tool of healing: the mind.

"It is your Father's good pleasure to give you the Kingdom." Luke 12:32

Empowerment or Guilt?

In my counseling of thousands of cancer patients, some would take this information in a negative fashion: "You mean I caused my own cancer?" This book is not about blame or guilt. It is about empowerment. Once you realize that you accidentally drove your car into a ditch, now it is time to get serious about careful driving. You are in charge. The

ONLY thing that we can control in this life is our thoughts. Make them healing thoughts.

Suggestions

Read the chapters on Healthy Pleasures and Inspiration From Geniuses. Each of these chapters has life changing information to shift your paradigm away from illness and toward wellness.

Thanksgiving

You cannot be grateful and unhappy at the same time. Start each day by saturating your mind with gratitude. If you are reading this book, then you have much to be thankful about in your everyday life, even if you have cancer.

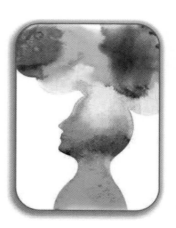

Forgiveness

Let it go. You are not endorsing the offense someone committed against you. You are merely "untying" them from you. You don't need to do lunch with them or ever see them again. Picture the offender climbing into a basket of a hot air balloon and being lifted gently up away out of sight, never to be seen by you again.

Seasoned meditators are able to shift their brain waves toward the more productive and healing alpha waves. You could practice meditation for 40 years before you get it right. Or you could pay $15,000 for an intensive 5 day workshop on biofeedback, <u>40 years of Zen</u>, to control your brain waves. Or you could just forgive everyone you can think of, which is one of the keys in biofeedback for shifting into healing alpha waves.

Meditation

The power of the mind can be focused, like a light can be focused into a laser. By stilling the mind you stop the endless flow of stress hormones that compound our health problems. Sit quietly for 20 minutes each day and simply focus on your breath as it flows across your nostrils.

Focus on a word or simply "breathing joy". While it is very difficult to shut down the mind, with training you can keep the mind in a state of peace, which encourages healing.

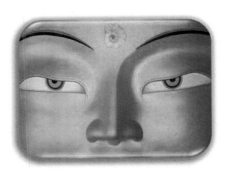

Go below the choppy waves of everyday mental chatter and experience the incredible tranquility that awaits you in the silence and the "space between your thoughts." There are many great websites that teach meditation as well as YouTube videos that demonstrate the process.[9] Search "I AM affirmations" on YouTube. Go to MindValley.com for uplifting education and inspirational videos.[10] Listen daily to the six phase meditation by Vishen Lakhiani on YouTube.[11] Saturate your mind with thoughts of wellness, happiness, joy and enthusiasm.

Creative Visualization

Picture your body the way you want it to be. Crowd out the disease with visions of health. Focus on that image for at least 30 minutes daily. Feel the feelings of being healthy, alive, alert, vibrant, and eager to address each new day. Since your mind is working all the time anyway, you might as well direct your mind toward thoughts of peace and healing as opposed to "awefulizing" about today and tomorrow.

Journaling

Write down your thoughts and feelings. Get detailed. No one will read this. You are not being charged for this. Express yourself starting wherever you are in your life. Journaling can be an amazing healing catharsis.

Belief System

What do you believe? About life? About yourself? What do you deserve? Do you think that illness means that people will pay attention to you? That you will not be expected to perform at a certain unrealistic standard? We have two computers running in our mind. The conscious mind makes efforts to decide daily activities. But the subconscious mind is 1 million times more powerful than the conscious mind and is driving the car. You can say all the affirmations you want about healing and wholeness, yet if your subconscious mind thinks that you deserve illness, or that illness will get other's attention, or that your doctor's prognosis that you will be dead in 2 years is accurate…then nothing can deter that belief system. Hypnosis attempts to access this subconscious mind to make radical changes in behavior, clearly demonstrated by the stage hypnotist who can make normal people do abnormal things. Emotional freedom technique (EFT), and eye movement desensitization reprocessing (EMDR) are other techniques that help reprogram the subconscious mind to be in harmony with your conscious goals.

Mental health begins with the statement: "I love myself." You cannot give away something that you do not have. Self-love does not mean narcissism. Self-love is an acceptance of yourself, an ability to stand in the mirror naked and say "you are fabulous, you have done a great job, you are perfect just as you are." Once you love yourself and can list reasons to be proud of yourself, then you can start giving love to others. But not until you start with yourself.

In the HEALING HEART [12] by Norman Cousins, the introduction by the director of cardiology at Harvard Medical School, speaks of a patient with severe cardiomyopathy (weak heart) where the attending physicians gathered around this doomed patient and one doctor spoke of a "sound gallop" in her heart beat.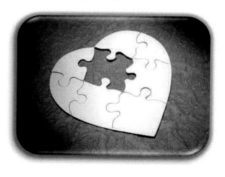
"Sound gallop" to the physicians meant that her heart beat was erratic and indicative of disease. "Sound gallop" to the patient created images of a strong horse eager to get on the racetrack. The patient got up and left and fully recovered after this doomsday diagnosis was spoken over her. Her belief system was the trump card in her healing.

Join a Group

Church, synagogue, mosque, AA, something. People who have the support of a clan do better in illness and wellness.

Find a Co-Patient

In working with thousands of cancer patients, I have found that those who have a helper, a co-patient, a friend, spouse, Rabbi, relative...someone who cares, who will take the cancer patient by the scruff of the neck and say "we are not quitting". Those cancer patients do better than those who are trying to summit the peak of Mt. Cancer by themselves.

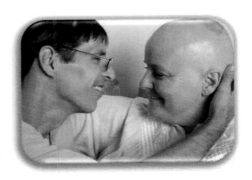

Sense of Purpose

On headstones in graveyards there is a birth date and death date that are separated by a dash. What are you doing with your "dash", or life? Fear of dying is not a sense of purpose. Get involved. Find a mission that you can believe in. Work, family, volunteer work, travel, community activist. Get your energies focused on a sense of purpose for your life.

BUT YOU'RE <u>STILL GONNA DIE</u>.[13]

"And the soul afraid of dying that never learns to live."
The Rose, by Bette Midler

Fear of death is not a reason to live. We are all going to die. There is a very entertaining song and video based on the <u>song by Shel Silverstein</u>. "You can jog up to heaven, but you're still gonna die. You can enroll in EST, get an AIDS test, move out west where it's sunny and dry...but you're still gonna die."

This acceptance of death is an important concept in this book on natural healing methods. There are some excellent books about people who have been clinically dead, then revived, then relate their experiences of death. Ray Moody, MD, PhD has a classic book LIFE AFTER LIFE in which he interviewed 150 people who were dead, then revived. Their stories are inspirational and informative of the "warmth and love" that greeted these people in death. Eben Alexander, MD was a Harvard based neurosurgeon, quasi-atheist who contracted an infection in his brain. His book, 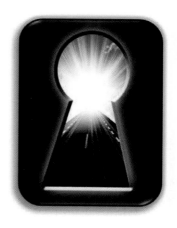 PROOF OF HEAVEN, has a moving and euphoric description of what our souls experience upon the transition of death. Dannion Brinkley wrote his SAVED BY THE LIGHT about his wonderful transformational experiences when dead. A beautiful country western song "The Dash" speaks of the dash that separates our birth and death years on our tombstone. What are you going to do with the dash?[14]

Let's hope that you will heal from your current health crisis. And by accepting death, the rest of your long and fruitful life will be even sweeter because you savor the moments and do not fear death.

Illness as a Teaching Tool

If we can get beyond the diagnosis of "cancer" and start thinking about "what is this crisis trying to teach me?" Many a cancer patient has stood at the podium of a celebrate life reunion and said "Cancer is the best thing that ever happened to me." When you recover your wits after this shocking statement, then the cancer victor will explain: "My life was not 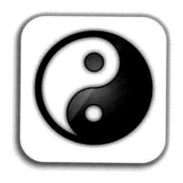 working. I did not appreciate myself or those around me. I needed to recalibrate my values. Cancer did that for me."

"Crisis" in Oriental language means "danger and opportunity". You have the opportunity to use cancer as a pole vault to bring your life to the next level. You can become a victor or a victim. Cancer can be the start of a new beginning in your life. A life filled with meaning, purpose, confidence, peace, joy, gratitude, love, kindness, generosity, and more. It's your call.

PATIENT PROFILE: BEAT END STAGE TUBERCULOSIS

True story. The number one cause of death throughout most of the 19th century was tuberculosis. Galen Clark went to Yosemite Valley to die of end stage tuberculosis at age 42 in the fall of 1856. His doctor told him that coughing up chunks of his lungs meant he had up to 2-6 months to live. There was no cure for this disease. Clark reasoned that "If I'm going to die soon, then I'm going to die in Yosemite, the prettiest place I've ever seen." He got happy. Scientists now tell us that happiness brings on the flow of endorphins, which supercharge our immune system and may slow down cancer.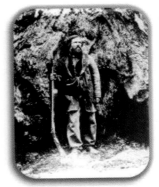

Next, Galen Clark carved his own tombstone, thus accepting his mortality, a ritual that would give us all a better appreciation of our finite time on earth. He then started eating what was available in Yosemite in those days; clean and lean wild game, mountain trout, nuts, berries, vegetables, and lots of clean water. No sugar and no dairy products. Lots of unplanned unavoidable intermittent fasting. He then began doing what he wanted to do, hiking and creating trails, in the place he treasured the most, Yosemite Valley. He didn't die 6 months later, but rather 54 years later, just shy of his 96th birthday. He bolstered his "non-specific host defense mechanisms" with good thoughts and good nutrition. You can do the same.

For more information about using your mind as the ultimate healing force go to GettingHealthier.com.

ENDNOTES

[1] https://www.cdc.gov/chronicdisease/about/costs/index.htm

[2] http://www.rehabchicago.org/the-human-brain/

[3] https://www.amazon.com/Reality-ESP-Physicists-Psychic-Abilities-ebook/dp/B00SKF0WLY/ref=sr_1_1?keywords=russell+targ&qid=1557755929&s=gateway&sr=8-1

[4] https://med.virginia.edu/perceptual-studies/

[5] https://www.heartmath.org/

[6] https://noetic.org/about/

[7] https://www.amazon.com/dp/B00DB3A1UC/ref=dp-kindle-redirect?_encoding=UTF8&btkr=1

[8] https://www.amazon.com/Mind-Over-Medicine-Lissa-Rankin-ebook/dp/B00BLSZJGA/ref=sr_1_2?crid=2S86YT71TGBN7&keywords=lissa+rankin&qid=1557797776&s=books&sprefix=lissa+rankin%2Caps%2C439&sr=1-2

[9] https://mindworks.org/blog/best-meditation-techniques-for-beginners/

[10] https://www.mindvalley.com/

[11] https://www.youtube.com/watch?v=oeQfRtiY-ZM

[12] https://www.amazon.com/Healing-Heart-Norman-Cousins/dp/0816136696

[13] https://www.youtube.com/watch?v=XQ2P4DKQ5ZI

[14] https://www.youtube.com/watch?v=m-NDCLgTUwU

KEY 4
ATTITUDE/THE MIND

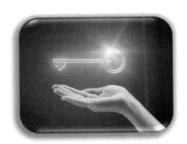

Chapter 4.1
Healthy Pleasures

FROM NATURE'S PHARMACY:
Healthy Fats That Make You Thin: EPA, GLA, CLA.

      Americans eat too much fat and the wrong kind of fat. Yet, there is equally convincing evidence that we have serious fatty acid deficiencies. Bad fats include hydrogenated, or trans fats, with no known safety level. Good fats include EPA from fish oil, GLA from borage or primrose oil, and CLA from the meat and milk of ruminant animals grazed on green grass. Each of these fats has merit in your diet and/or supplement program. According to Andrew Stoll, MD of Harvard, fish oil may prevent or reverse early stages of heart disease, dysplasias (pre-cancerous conditions), depression, auto-immune disease (like multiple sclerosis and arthritis), diabetes, skin problems, and obesity. GLA is a powerful anti-inflammatory fat. CLA was a true surprise for the researchers when they found that something in hamburger could have anti-cancer activity. When ruminants (cows, sheep, deer, buffalo, etc.) eat green grass, the linoleic acid (which promotes cancer) in the stomach is converted to conjugated linoleic acid, which has been shown to slow or delay cancer and may reduce fat deposits in humans. Grass fed animals have 500% more CLA than grain fed animals.

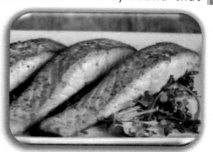

Too many people have a misunderstanding about a healthy lifestyle. People get the notion that everything they like is forbidden and everything they are supposed to eat tastes awful. While watching hours of TV and having a bowl of ice cream might give you a few moments of immediate gratification, the long-term consequences are full of pain and discomfort. The unhealthy lifestyle eventually leads to medication, disability, pain, depression, surgeries, and long waits in doctors' offices.

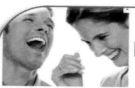

HEALTHY PLEASURES

WHOLE FOODS	FRIENDSHIPS
DARK CHOCOLATE	SUNSHINE
NAPS/SIESTA	HOT SAUCE
RED WINE	MUSIC
LAUGHTER	VACATIONS
SEX	PRAYER/MED.
WALKS	THANKSGIV.
MEANINGFUL WORK	

The healthy lifestyle not only remedies the above situations, but also has immediate gratification, as you will see below. All of these modalities feel good and are scientifically proven to bolster your health. While not all of these healthy pleasures may be possible for you right now, keep them in mind for when they are practical. Our strategy in this book is to engage all of your healing faculties into a grand symphony of wellness that cannot be denied. The more wellness you have in your body, the less illness you can have in your body. What are you waiting for! Have fun and get well.

Laughter

"Humor is the balancing stick that allows us to walk the tightrope of life." John Kennedy, 35th president USA

History is rich in the primitive attempts of our ancestors to reap the benefits of laughter. Ancient kings would employ the court jester to make him laugh. Humor is fooling the mind, with an unexpected punch line. Humor allows us to tolerate the injustices and incongruities of life. The logical mind struggles with the problems of life. The humorous mind provides shock absorbers to better tolerate the undesirable aspects of life.

The TV show MASH was one of the longest running shows in TV history, spanning 1972-83 and 256 episodes. It was more than great casting, acting, and script writing that propelled this success. The MASH episodes were about draftees in Korea around 1950 who were trying to make the most out of an intolerable situation. Stuck 8000 miles from home in a hostile situation with death all around, the MASH team did their best to keep a sense of humor, which make the macabre setting tolerable. We can all learn something from the MASH TV shows.

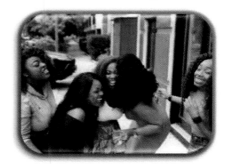

Hunter Campbell, MD opened a free hospital in 1971 with humor and dignity as its primary goals for the patients. The 1998 movie Patch Adams highlighted this dedicated doctor and his use of humor in a setting of sickness. Norman Cousins used humor to help reverse his arthritic condition and later his heart attack. His books, ANATOMY OF AN ILLNESS and THE HEALING HEART are classic works of the link between the health of the mind and the body. Cousins called laughter "internal jogging".

What do the following longevity experts have in common?
Answer: All are comedians who outlived their peers by a decade or so.

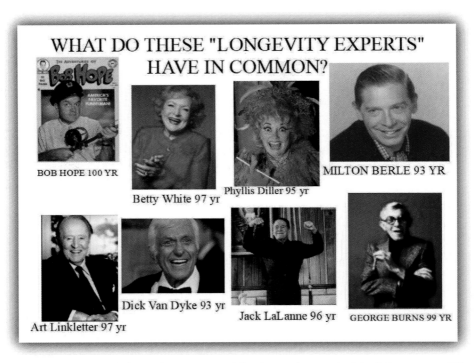

We could inundate you with the science behind humor. There are <u>wonderful organizations</u>[1] and websites that have documented the peer reviewed science behind <u>laughter and health</u>. We could show you the clear evidence linking depression with heart disease, cancer, Alzheimer's and more. We could show you how there are measurable changes in the immune panel and digestion of someone who had a good laugh.

Or we could just turn you loose on YouTube.com and let you chuckle your way through the thousands of great humor videos available for free. Search for Jerry Seinfeld, Dean Martin Celebrity Roasts, Larry the Cable Guy, Kathleen Madigan, Jeff Foxworthy, or any of the other talented comedians online. Remember, don't take yourself too seriously. None of us are getting out of this life alive. Have fun. Wag more, bark less.

Dance
"Let them praise His name with dancing." Psalms 149:3
"Dance like no one is watching."

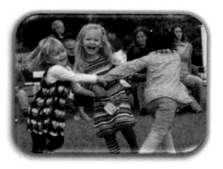

Most human cultures throughout all of history have included dance in their celebrations. Dance is innate in the human brain and body. Watch a 2 year old child listening to music. You can't stop them from dancing. Somehow we lose that pizzazz for dance as we age. Men start looking at dance as though it is not manly. Most people do not take ballroom dance lessons and hence feel incompetent on the dance floor. But when you watch a couple who really know how to dance, there is magic in the air. Two people move effortlessly as one unit, what is called murmurations in the animal kingdom. Ever watch a school of fish or flock of birds moving as one unit? How do they do that? That is what human dance can be like. Poetry in motion. And it is not just graceful, dance is a powerful therapeutic agent.

The scientific studies are proving the health merits of ballroom dancing. Ballroom dancing at least once per week has been shown to reduce the risk of Alzheimer's disease by 73%. Nothing else came close to this level of efficacy. If dancing was a patentable drug, then the good news about its health benefits would be broadcast throughout media and the internet.

Not to be pedantic or an elitist, but line dancing and free form movement to electronic dance music does not have the same benefits as learning the skills of ballroom dancing, coordinating the two hemispheres of the brain with music as the conductor, holding a partner's hand and body. Use it or lose it. Dancing stimulates neuroplasticity to encourage nerve pathways that maintain our mental and physical health. Dancing is a surmountable challenge, which is one of the key criteria for our own happiness. In the classical bestseller FLOW, the author explains the link between a surmountable (doable, but not easy) challenge and happiness.

Check out your local websites for dance studios. Check out DanceVision.com for their extensive line of videos to help you learn to dance. There are about 30 different dances, including waltz, foxtrot, rhumba, tango, etc; each of which is taught at bronze, silver, then gold levels. You will never get bored learning to dance. And you may avoid disability through weekly dancing.

Get a pair of dancing shoes. Find a partner or group to join. Use a dance instructor. In the beginning of your lessons, you may feel awkward. That's normal. Persist. Within months you will be using a therapy, dancing, that is so powerful in its healing abilities that it must be listed somewhere in a hospital formulary.

Play Music
"We are giving birth to God's children."
Ludwig van Beethoven on creating music

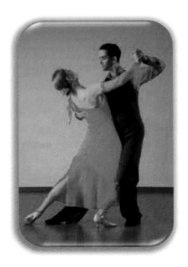

At the tail end of my high school years, a friend, Mike Partin, showed me the chords to the House of the Rising Sun on my uncle's borrowed guitar. I was hooked. Within two years of playing guitar, I was entertaining professionally in bars. Then I decided playing music was a waste of time and I needed to concentrate on my career. My guitar got tucked into its case for a long winter's nap of 20 years or so. Then I discovered the textbook from the New York

Academy of Sciences <u>THE BIOLOGICAL FOUNDATIONS OF MUSIC</u>, in which these academically affiliated authors found substantial changes in the human brain when playing a musical instrument.[2]

"Playing a musical instrument unmasks existing but inoperative neuronal pathways."

In other words, playing music opens up "freeways" in your brain. I went back to my guitars, then added the piano later. I am never bored and have no time for TV. There are infinite opportunities for playing music. It reduces stress. It enhances a sense of joy and wellness.

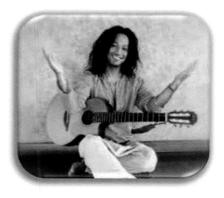

Today's modern musician is exposed to a Pandora's box of dangerous enticements: alcohol, tobacco, drugs, late nights, and poor lifestyle habits. Which explains why musicians of that category die sooner than normal. Yet, the concert trained musician actually has a healthier and longer life than normal people. When a major university examined the lifespan of faculty members, the music department had the longest longevity.

Playing a musical instrument can be as simple and affordable as a harmonica or ukulele; or can stretch anyone's capacity through learning the piano or violin. The joys of learning to play a musical instrument cannot be overstated. The <u>health benefits</u> are well documented. Let the concert of your life begin.

Listen to Music
"I'm pickin' up good vibrations." Good Vibrations, the Beach Boys

It's all about vibrations. All of the sciences can eventually be boiled down to vibrations. All of life vibrates. Some of those vibrations we can see as light and color. Some of those vibrations we can hear as sound. Most vibrations can be neither seen nor heard. Here is where music starts looking like the <u>medicine of the 21st century</u>. Music therapists have proven that music can change moods, heart rate, immune functions, digestion, alertness and more.

All religious ceremonies throughout all of time have involved music. Chanting, singing, musical instruments all became the warm up act for connecting with the Divine. Some of the most inspired music in our human spectrum was written through the supernatural feelings of religious celebrations, such as Christmas.

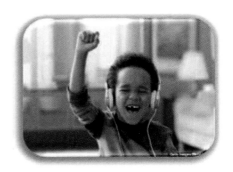

Among the many benefits of listening to music for the cancer patient are included: <u>stress reduction,</u> better sleep, enhanced mood. Music can help cancer patients better tolerate the rigors of chemo and radiation therapy. You can listen to nearly any song or any genre of music via internet radio, such as Pandora and Amazon music, or watch the performers do their musical magic on YouTube.com.

Arts and Crafts

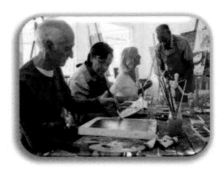

People have been painting, carving, and humming since the dawn of time. Humans are artistic people who appreciate creativity. Pick a craft: painting, sewing, needle work, calligraphy, weaving, photography, pottery, wood carving, etc. The health benefits of crafts are so profound that many hospitals and nursing homes have an activity director to help steer people in the right direction. <u>Health benefits</u> of arts and crafts include stress relief, confidence boost, improve empathy, improves quality of life for those with illness, boosts brain productivity, lessen effect of serious health conditions. The <u>American Journal of Public Health</u> includes a peer reviewed article on The Connection Between Art, Healing, and Public

Health. Pick out some fun craft and take a class or study on YouTube.com.

Sex

"We are all born sexual creatures, thank God, but it's a pity so many people despise and crush this natural gift." Marilyn Monroe

Sex feels good. That's why there are 7.7 billion people on earth. The mental and physical health benefits of sex are dazzling:

- Improves sleep
- Augments immune functions
- Reduces risk for prostate cancer
- Elevates heart rate for cardiovascular workout
- Improves libido
- Reduces risk of incontinence in women
- Lowers blood pressure
- Reduces pain
- Lowers risk for heart attack
- Improves sense of well being
- Burns calories
- Relieves stress
- Improves intimacy and relationships (via oxytocin)
- Improves appearance (via estrogen and testosterone)
- Improves lifespan.

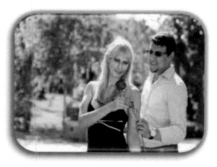

For decades researchers have been trying to better understand the benefits of sex. In a decade long study of 1000 middle aged men, those who had the most orgasms had one half the death rate compared to fewer orgasms. You already have your own ideas of morality on sex. Sex between consenting adults can be a beautiful and healthy experience for both partners. If you are deep into cancer treatment, then sex may not be possible, but cuddling with a loved one or even a pet can provide that tactile sense of being with another being.

Walks

The benefits of exercise are astounding. No drug comes close to the risk to benefit to cost ratio of a good walk. You probably will not be weightlifting or playing soccer until the day before you die, but you likely could take a walk the day before you die. Some people use ear buds from their smartphone and listen to music or uplifting recordings. Some people consider a walk in nature to be a moving meditation. Try silence while walking. Try meditating while walking. Brisk walking, or "wogging" is a great way to get you up to target heart rate. While walking with a partner or pet is nice, you do not need a companion. You can walk in nearly any weather. Just need a decent pair of shoes.

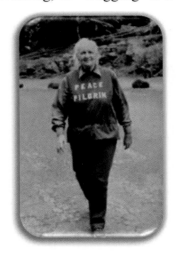

Think of Peace Pilgrim, a middle age woman who sold and gave away everything, brought nothing with her, and walked over 25,000 miles as a peace activist and vegan before she stopped counting the miles. She died at age 72 as a passenger in a rare car ride, but her mental and physical health were decades younger than her age. Walking is a panacea.

Meditation
"You've mastered the selfie. Now master thyself." Unknown

The human mind is the most remarkable device/machine/entity on earth. Even the most erudite neurosurgeon will speak with humility about the functions and potential of the human brain. Mystics for many millennia have discovered the secret to preserving the mind: meditation. Seasoned meditators have demonstrated an ability to control functions of the body that scientists thought were on automatic pilot, such as heart rate, blood pressure, and basal metabolism.

Meditation dates back to 5000 BCE (before common era) and continued its spread and evolution through various religions and philosophies until the 1960s when great teachers from Asia came to the West to train people in meditation. Harvard professor Herbert Benson, MD found in 1967 that there were measurable benefits from meditation. The Beatles studied meditation in India to help deal with the stress of their overwhelming fame and fortune.

Again, thinking of a risk to benefit to cost ratio, nothing comes close to meditation. The science-based benefits of meditation makes any drug developer drool with envy:

- Reduces stress
- Controls anxiety
- Promotes emotional health
- Enhances self-awareness
- Lengthens attention span
- Generates kindness
- Fight addictions
- Improves sleep
- Controls pain
- Decreases blood pressure
- Slows cognitive decline or memory loss

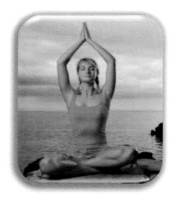

There are many forms of meditation: silence, chanting, listen to repetitious music, stare at a candle or mandela, repeat a prayer, repeat a mantra, variations on self-hypnosis, etc. You can follow any of the guided meditations on YouTube, such as the 6 phase meditation by Vishen Lakhiani.[3]

Here are the very basic elements of meditation: sit quietly in a quiet area where you will not be disturbed. Close your eyes. Begin deep belly breathing and clear your mind. Focus on the breath as it moves past the rim of your nostrils. Slow your breathing to long deep diaphragm breaths. As you inhale, picture the air as perfect white light filling your body. As you exhale, picture yourself glowing with white light. Set aside at least 20 minutes daily for this ritual that will leave you relaxed and energized at the same time. Meditation feels good, costs nothing, you can do it anywhere, and has tremendous benefits. There is no downside here.

Altruism: Helping Others

"Every man must decide whether he will walk in the light of creative altruism or in the darkness of destructive selfishness."
Dr. Martin Luther King, Jr.

Humans have a war going on inside of us. Our ego wants/demands attention and everything now. Our ego wants to be the center of everything. Our ego seeks self-preservation without concern for others. We also have a conscience or soul with morals and values that include empathy. The human species survived this long by living in groups or clans, which means we give up some of our ego tantrums and must yield to the betterment of the clan.

Ego says "keep all the money, you might need it someday". The soul says "what if kindness were a religion and we shared with each other". Ego says "every man for himself" while the soul says "how can I reduce the suffering of others". In the gut wrenching and international bestselling book <u>MAN'S SEARCH FOR MEANING</u> Dr. Victor Frankl, a neurologist and psychiatrist and survivor of 4 Nazi concentration camps, found that the people who survived these intolerable conditions often developed a sense of compassion, control, and altruism. Imagine giving a piece of your bread to another when you are also starving.

<u>Altruism is good</u> for your physical and mental health. Tithe (ten percent) your income to a <u>worthy charity</u>. Volunteer your time and talents to the needy. The story is told of a person who died and in the afterlife was shown a large banquet room ornately decorated and filled with people sitting at a long banquet table that was overflowing with delightful food. Only problem was that the people were given forks that were too long to feed themselves. Everyone was frustrated with this banquet that they could not partake. "What is this?" asked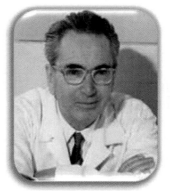

the person to his/her guide. "Hell". Across the hall from this scene was an identical scene in which the people were feeding each other with the same long forks. "This is heaven."

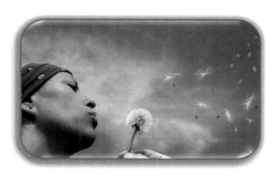

Feed each other. Help those less fortunate than you. Teach a person how to fish, but you might need to give them a fish until they learn the skill. Everyone benefits in the process.

Journal Writing

Long ago, before oxygen, TV, and the internet were invented, people did something else with their time. The first efforts at writing were journaling. Since then, psychologists have documented the <u>83 benefits of journaling</u>. Journaling allows you to gather your thoughts into a cohesive fashion. Journaling allows you to vomit your emotions on something that eagerly takes the anger, fear, depression, and deepest thoughts. Your journal never judges you or charges you. Most of our early history comes from journals from famous explorers, leaders, scientists. Yet, you do not have to be famous to derive exceptional benefits from journaling. Costs nearly nothing, no downside, takes little time, and make you a happier and healthier person.

Forgiveness

"An eye for an eye and the whole world is blind."
Mahatma Gandhi.

Anger and vengeance are like swallowing acid and expecting it to hurt the person you hate. By forgiving, you do not endorse the person's act against you, you merely move on. The Lord's Prayer from the <u>original Aramaic version</u> says: "untie the knots of failure binding us". When you forgive, you untie the person who injured you. You release them. You let them go their way. Their punishment will come. Let the Universe take care of that.

Psychologists consider forgiveness to be the "queen" of emotional health. There are many peer reviewed articles documenting the <u>health benefits of forgiveness</u>. "Chronic <u>unforgiving may erode health</u> whereas forgiving responses may enhance it."

Louise Hay (see chapter on Inspiration from Geniuses) was a victim by many people throughout her life, including rape as a young girl. Louise was diagnosed with cancer and decided to change her thoughts and her life. She forgave her transgressors. Doesn't mean she condoned their behavior or wanted to have lunch with them. She merely untied them from her life.

The <u>Forty Years of Zen</u> program teaches people through biofeedback how to harness their thoughts and enhance happiness, health, and productivity.[4] These researchers have found that the best way to upgrade your alpha brain waves is to forgive…everybody, completely. Watch your life take off. Picture your enemy/teacher climbing into a hot air balloon basket and you cut the cord so they float away. They are gone from your life.

Friendships

After spending billions of dollars and thousands of hours from brilliant researchers, the National Institutes of Health concluded that the <u>biggest risk factor for heart disease</u> is loneliness. Humans are social creatures. Isolation and loneliness may be acceptable for some personality types, but in general loneliness kills. Build a social network of friends. Social media does not count. Texting someone is not the same as taking a walk or sharing a cup of tea with a friend. Pets can be great friends. Use some of the websites, like <u>Meetup.com</u>, to find people of like interests and values. Someone out there needs you as a friend.

Beauty and Nature

"Allow nature's peace to flow into you as sunshine flows into trees."
John Muir, father of Yosemite and Sequoia National Parks

There is beauty all around us. Any season, any place on earth has some beauty to it. You see more of what you focus on. While the average American looks at a screen (TV, computer, cell phone) for 10 hours per day, by taking a few of those hours and immersing yourself in nature, you may find a whole new level of peace. There is <u>compelling evidence</u> that surrounding oneself in nature can be healing. <u>Feng shui</u> is an ancient Chinese art that uses the elements of nature (water, flowers, trees, wood, chimes, wind) to create a harmonious atmosphere in your home or workplace. Immerse yourself in beauty to the maximum extent of your schedule. You

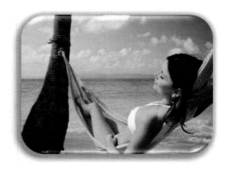

may find art galleries areas of inspiration. You might like wood carving exhibits. Go for the beauty. You will be happier and more relaxed and begin a mysterious process of healing within.

Chocolate
"When it comes to chocolate, resistance is futile."
Regina Brett

Over 4000 years ago, brown food prepared from the cacao seeds was being used by Aztec and Maya people in Mexico and Central America. Since chocolate contains small amounts of caffeine, it was assumed throughout the 1970s through 2000 that chocolate must be bad for our health. While any food will have an adverse reaction for a certain segment of the population,

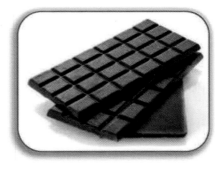

chocolate appears to be well tolerated. So well tolerated that the world consumes over 7 million metric tons per year with Europeans the world champion in consumption.

Then researchers isolated flavonoids in chocolate and began doing some epidemiological studies on people who ate a lot of chocolate. What they found brought a round of applause from the Willie Wonka fans. Dark <u>chocolate is rich in</u> flavonoids, procyanidins, and antioxidants that are very good for your health. Have some dark chocolate chips (60%

cacao and above) or chocolate bars on a regular basis, and <u>your body will thank you</u> for it.

Red Wine
"I cook with wine. Sometimes I even add it to the food." W.C. Fields

Wild chimps in Guinea have been observed creating a sponge from leaves then <u>regularly consuming alcohol</u> palm wine. Primates seem to favor "happy hours". "It's a medicine and a poison," states Brad Paisley's song "<u>Alcohol</u>", which is a classic video on YouTube.com. Alcohol, in general, has caused more deaths, more divorces, more domestic violence than nearly any conceivable provocateur. Which is why several religions ban alcohol and the USA tried to ban alcohol during the Prohibition years of 1920-1933. Didn't work. Alcohol consumption went up, the feds went broke trying to break up stills and the Mafia was born on this black market product. That said, the difference between a medicine and a poison is dosage. Let's talk about that.

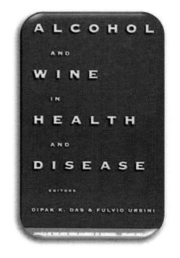

You need protein, but not too much or you tax the kidneys and liver and create a metabolic acidosis. You need fiber, but not too much or you generate indigestion and diarrhea. The data on modest consumption of alcohol clearly points to health benefits. And the best of the alcohols is red wine, possibly due to the resveratrol content, which seems to protect cells. Academically affiliated researchers reporting in the <u>peer reviewed journal</u> Annual Review of Nutrition state:

"individuals with the habit of daily moderate wine consumption enjoy significant reductions in all-cause and particularly cardiovascular mortality"

Red wine seems to help generate more dopamine in the body, which is good. We are only beginning to grasp the health impact of red wine as over 9000 flavonoids have been identified and several are in red wine, which shows beneficial effects on the microbiota in the gut. Some studies have found a link between alcohol consumption and breast cancer. However, the famous Framingham study looked at alcohol intake among 5000 women over the course of 24-48 years and found no link between alcohol and breast cancer.

The New York Academy of Sciences has compiled a textbook: ALCOHOL AND WINE IN HEALTH AND DISEASE which shows the overwhelming data on health benefits of modest alcohol consumption. The Report on Sensible Drinking from the Department of Health in the United Kingdom actually suggested:

"...may wish to consider the possibility that light drinking might benefit their health."

And you say "that's fine for normal people, but what about us cancer patients?" I have counseled many cancer patients who told me of their nightly ritual with their mate sharing a glass of wine and discussing the day's events. I suggested that these people continue their happy hour. Many of them recovered from their cancer. The stress of changing a highly cherished ritual may be more harmful than a small amount of alcohol. Alcoholics and pregnant women should not drink. After that, it's up to you and your doctor.

Meaningful Work
"Work like you don't need the money." Unknown

When Social Security was first implemented in the US in 1935 the average life expectancy was 61 years and retirement was put at 65 years. You do the math. The Social Security Administration did not expect to be providing for so many people for so long. We now see that meaningful work is associated with higher income and longer life. In the classic book FLOW, the author shows that happiness comes from being in the present moment and having a surmountable challenge, aka meaningful work.

The human mind is so bright and the spirit so eager that it needs to have a direction for these energies. You don't need to earn a paycheck in your work. It could be volunteer work. It could be a craft that you donate to charity raffles. Humans without a sense of purpose are like a ship without a rudder, just drifting. "Figure out something you would do for free, then find a way to get paid to do it." Great advice for a happier and healthier person.

Naps

The cynic claims that real people only sleep when it is dark outside. But not so fast. Many Latin and European countries have made siesta time a 3 hour national holiday every day. Now we find that there are dramatic benefits to napping, including sleep quality and mental health. R,searchers have even gone so far as to pinpoint

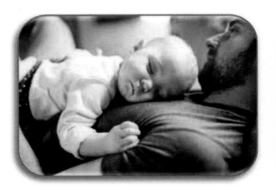

the sweet spot in napping, somewhere between 10 and 30 minutes, restores wakefulness and enhances performance. More than 30 minutes of napping seems to retard performance and induce drowsiness.

No one is more in need of their faculties than airline pilots. So airlines provide separate sleeping quarters where pilots on long flights might spend half of the flight in slumberland. So get out your soother or white noise device, put on your sleep mask, and revitalize your body for 30 minutes in the afternoon.

Sleep

While napping in the afternoon is not practical for some people, sleeping, especially at night, is mandatory for all. Most people in advanced society stagger around in a state of chronic sleep deprivation. This is extremely bad for mental and physical health. In one study

<u>researchers</u> took away 3 hours each night from 12 subjects in the sleep lab. The subjects were not only sleepier, but had impaired psychomotor performance, but even more surprising they had elevations in inflammation (proinflammatory cytokines). Inflammation is the beginning of most degenerative diseases, including heart disease and cancer. Researchers found that nearly <u>all categories of mental performance</u>, including interpersonal skills, declined radically with sleep deprivation. <u>Sleep deprivation</u> has been associated with decline in immune functions and elevation in inflammation. Sleep deprivation <u>decreased insulin sensitivity</u>, which will bring about a cascade of negative health effects. There is

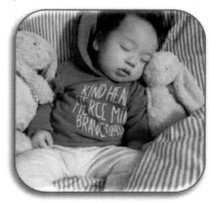

substantial evidence that night shift work (aka graveyard) <u>increases the risk for cancer</u>. If you do swing shift, then rotate with others for day shift on occasion. The more hours of light at night, the greater the risk for cancer in night shift workers.

According to some experts, the diseases of civilization expanded dramatically with the invention of the electric light bulb by Thomas Edison. Prior to the bulb, people generally went to bed when it got dark out. With the light bulb, people could stay up, thus promoting sleep deprivation.

Get a good night's sleep. It feels good and it is as essential as vitamins and water. If you have problems sleeping, try the nutrition supplements of L-tryptophan, GABA, melatonin, 5HTP, lavender, CBD, cannabis (if legal in your area). There are many excellent applications for your smartphone that can help put you to sleep. Before you drift off to sleep, program your mind with what you want to happen in your life. See images of your dreams coming true, give thanks for them, then drift off to a pleasant slumber.

Vacations

Global tourism is an <u>$8 trillion/yr business</u>, making it one of the largest and fastest growing industries on the planet. And there are good reasons. Vacations make you feel better and enhance general mental and physical health. There are many <u>proven benefits to regular vacations</u>. Researchers find that vacationers show benefits from stress reduction with fewer complaints of headache, back ache, heart irregularities and had a prolonged effect 5 weeks after the vacation.

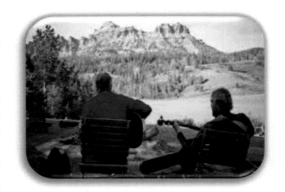

Because of the stress reduction and the link between stress and heart attacks, researchers found that people who skipped their vacations five years in a row were 30% more likely to have a heart attack. Improved productivity and better sleep rounded out the health benefits of vacations.

You don't have to spend a lot of money on a vacation. "Staycations" have become popular. Meaning, stay near your home. Do something different. Go somewhere different. Do not work while vacationing. Put away the smart devices. Chill out. Have some fun. Get healthier.

Exercise

"Does refusing to go to the gym count as resistance training?"

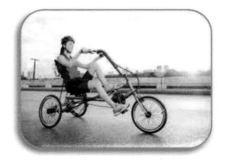

We have become a sedentary society. 2/3 of Americans are overweight and, obviously, 2/3 of Americans admit to no exercise. See the chapter on exercise for more information. We are under exercising ourselves to death. You have to use it or you will lose it. Car manufacturers have an interesting clause in their warranty: the car must be driven or the warranty is null and void. That goes for your body, too.

We are not talking about extreme exercises. While we all admire long distance runners, many of them develop musculoskeletal problems. Better yet, do something fun, like biking. There are biking trails all over the country to make biking a bed and breakfast extravaganza. Or dancing. Ballroom dancing puts a smile on everyone's face. Or pickleball, a cross between ping pong, badminton, and tennis. Lots of fun.

<u>Dis-ease may be from dis-use of the body</u>, advises Stanford physician Walter Bortz, MD.[5]

Gardening
"To plant a garden is to believe in tomorrow."

There are miracles going on all around us if we merely take the time to notice. How does a tomato seed, the size of a BB become a plant

the size of a man, then produce hundreds of tomato fruit, which each include dozens of seeds for future generations? To garden is to touch the Divine. Nourishing plants whether for beauty or consumption is a connection with the Keeper of the Universe

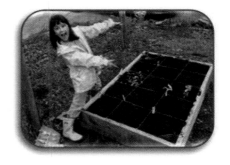

Gardening has many proven health benefits to mind and body. Gardens are now being <u>added to hospitals</u> and clinics for their healing value. Gardens have been added to <u>thousands of schools</u> across the country for their value in education and cooperative teamwork. Eating what you grow is a true spiritual experience. <u>Community gardens</u> not only provide stress reduction, healthy food, and outdoor activities, but also nourish a sense of connection with others.

You might consider the topic of <u>EDIBLE LANDSCAPING</u>, which means "why spend time and money growing a lawn when you can grow something that you can eat." According to NASA, there are about 49,000 square miles (128,000 square kilometers) of lawns that are mowed often in the USA. Maybe that time, money, gas, and water could be better spent on edible landscaping.

You could start small with your garden. A potted plant, or milkweed to attract butterflies, or a dwarf tree, or a succulent garden. Gardening is good for your body, mind, and spirit, and the planet.

Praise and Worship

"The closer you get to the truth, the clearer becomes the beauty and the more you will find worship welling up within you."
N.T.Wright

When the hard core scientist and physician Hans Selye, MD started his research in 1956 on the physiological effects of stress, he had no idea where his <u>research would lead him</u>. Selye, who was nominated for the Nobel prize in medicine 17 times, ultimately wrote about <u>attitude changes</u> that could minimize stress in modern society. Selye found stress reduction in 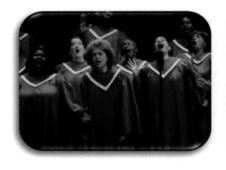 "altruistic egotism", that is, helping others with the anticipation of eventually helping yourself in the process. And "lean on a Higher Power", that is stop trying to micromanage a complex universe. On the dollar bill, the founding fathers of America wrote "In God we trust". They were mirroring the words of Selye and many brilliant philosophers before and since.

We live in a vast universe. The latest guess is that the universe is about 13.7 billion years old and thus 27 billion light years in diameter. If you want to read about LIFE AFTER LIFE, try Dr. Ray Moody's book on 150 case studies of people who were clinically dead, then reported to Dr. Moody their experiences of life after life. Or read any of the emerging books on quantum physics, which dazzles even the bright minds. Suffice it to say that there are many mysteries in our universe. One way to limit our stress in this skull cracking puzzle of life is to "lean on a Higher

Power". When you think of a Power that is everywhere throughout all of eternity, worship is the next move.

There has long been a link between faith, religion, and health. Studies have found that attending regular spiritual services may reduce mortality by 55%. If worship was a patentable drug, it would be a blockbuster. There have been unlimited cases of spontaneous healing in people who attended spiritual healing services. Faith in a better tomorrow, trust in a Supreme Being, belief in the afterlife, tolerance, kindness, patience, forgiveness, charity...these are the tenets of most religions. All of this is good for body, mind, and spirit.

Thanksgiving
You cannot be grateful and unhappy at the same time.

Gratitude or thanksgiving is a hallmark of mental health. The human mind is built for survival, to see the lion hiding in the tall grass, to look for trouble. But that survival mechanism can become our downfall if we only spot the blemishes in life. GRATITUDE: A WAY OF LIFE by Louise Hay was a life-changing book for me.

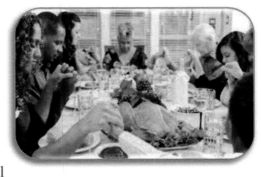

When you begin to count your blessings, when you see the miracles around you, when you develop a sense of thanksgiving for everything you get, have, do...then you are in a state of bliss. Which is exactly what you want in order to optimize mental and physical health. Gratitude is recognized by professional psychologists as a therapeutic intervention for mental health recovery.

Start every day with a lengthy list of reasons to be grateful. Take regular breaks throughout the day for the same exercise. You and everyone around you will see a noticeable change in your demeanor.

Sunshine
"Sunshine on my shoulders makes me happy." John Denver

93 million miles away from earth there is a magnificent thermonuclear fireball that is 109 times the size of earth…the sun. Every second, 600 million tons of hydrogen are fused into helium to generate a surface temperature of 10,000 F (5600 C) or 27 million F at the core. The sun's rays are carcinogenic, mutagenic, ionizing radiation such as was emitted at the atomic blast of Hiroshima. And the sun is the beginning of life on earth. Nearly all forms of life require light and infrared heat.

Then we come back to the invaluable aphorism: "The difference between a medicine and a poison is dosage." Former NASA researcher has written a well documented book on **EMBRACE THE SUN** to better understand the science behind rational sun exposure. Most modern humans are deprived of their rational dose of ultraviolet rays. A Harvard 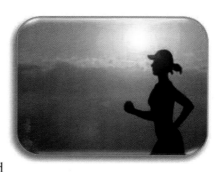 researcher with colleagues have written a textbook on the therapeutic uses of the various frequencies of light to heal many conditions in **PHOTOBIOMODULATION**. There is overwhelming evidence that some people are deeply affected by lack of sunlight in the winter, aka seasonal affective disorder, or winter depression.

Excess sunlight is a major contributor to basal and squamous cell cancers of the skin. Yet the lowest incidence of melanoma, the most lethal form of skin cancer, is found in outdoor workers.[6] Sunlight upon the skin not only generates vitamin D, which is a powerful anti-cancer substance and regulates 20% of the human genome, but also works as ultraviolet blood irradiation in activating the immune system through the veins which are closest to the surface of the skin.

"Outdoor work exposure seemed to have little effect on the risk of melanoma."

according to researchers published in the International Journal of Cancer. Since the most common melanomas are found on areas of skin that receive less sun, experts have postulated that melanoma is a collision between a bad sunburn on fair skin combined with a collapse of the immune system.

<u>Researchers have noted that</u>:

"sun exposure may also improve outcome from cancers of the breast, colon and prostate and Hodgkin lymphoma."

How can we explain the difference here. Is sun good or bad for humans? Think of our ancestors. They spent most of their waking hours outside. In northern climates, these people might start working outdoors in March and slowly build a tan that would protect the body from cancer. Today, we spend 9 months of the winter inside, then charge outside in June to get a bad sunburn. We take dark skin people, tell them to wear a suit to work, stay inside all year, then wonder why African Americans have a higher than normal incidence of obesity, diabetes, breast and prostate cancers, and more. Dark skinned people need more sun to get the same benefits as fair skin people. African Americans have a **very high incidence of vitamin D deficiency**.[7] Sun is not the problem. Sun is part of the solution. A tan is good. A burn is bad. Any questions?

Skin

The 9600 dermatologists in the USA treat nearly 5 million adults annually for skin cancers. But sunshine is not the only culprit here. **Antioxidants from fruits and vegetables** have been shown to significantly lower the risk for skin cancer. The most commonly eaten fruits and vegetables in America are catsup, French fries, and onion rings; which do little to lower the risk for skin cancer. It is our "weekend warrior" approach to sun that gives us trouble. Tuberculosis, which killed 14% of the global population for centuries, was due, **in part to avoiding the sun**.

Michael Hollick, MD, PhD is not only a physician but one of the principle researchers on vitamin D. Dr. Hollick's book on the value of sunshine **THE UV ADVANTAGE** got him fired from his position in the department of dermatology at Boston University. Rational exposure to sunlight will generate vitamin D, regulate the immune system through ultraviolet blood irradiation, help generate melatonin for anti-aging and sleep enhancement.

Eyes

For centuries, sailors were known for developing "ophthalmia", a condition of inflammation of the eyes, for staring at the reflection of the sun on the water. Eskimos created their own "sun glasses" by carving a narrow slit in bones or shells joined together to protect themselves from snow blindness. The eyes, especially blue eyes, can be damaged by excessive sun. However, our ancestors spent most of their waking hours outside. From that exposure our eyes developed a need for irrigating the eyes with indirect sunlight.

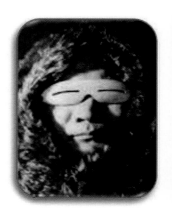

William Bates, MD was an opthalmologist in the 1920s in the US who published his book THE CURE OF IMPERFECT SIGHT BY TREATMENT WITHOUT GLASSES. A cornerstone of the Bates program was exposing the eyes to indirect sunlight. Optometrist and researcher Jacob Liberman has written an excellent book on the therapeutic value of sunlight and the various frequencies within sunlight to heal many ailments including poor vision.

BOTTOM LINE. Protect your eyes. Use hat and sunglasses when in very bright situations. When outside and there is no glare, allow your naked eyes to absorb the healing energies of full spectrum sunlight.

Touching
"Your hand touching mine. This is how galaxies collide."
Sanober Khan

Humans have five main senses: taste, smell, vision, hearing, and touch. That sense of touch protects us from being burned or frozen. Touch can give us great pleasure. And touch is an essential nutrient, just as much as water. Researchers have conducted experiments with babies in which both groups were given all their nutrient needs, but one group was denied touch. The touch less group experienced weight loss and became sickly.

Therapeutic massage and healing touch have been shown to improve symptoms in cancer patients being medically treated, with measurable reductions in pain, mood disturbance, and fatigue. Urban legend says that Bob Hope credited daily massages with one of the reasons that he lived well until 100. Perhaps one of the reasons that pet owners have better health is the touch they get with their pets. The benefits of dance include touching another person. Try healing touch, or massage, or cuddling, or hugs when appropriate.

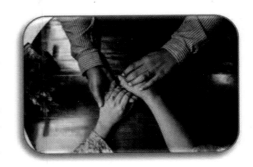

PATIENT PROFILE

A.J. was diagnosed in 2014 with mesothelioma, aka asbestiosis. A.J. had been given a very poor prognosis by his doctors. He had a consultation with PQ in May 2, 2016, and PQ was the first medical professional to give him hope. As a result of PQs recommendations he has subsequently seen an oncologist and family doctors specializing in functional and integrative medicine. A.J. believes nutrition has played a major part in his recovery. Since his consultation with PQ, he now eats a clean diet, mostly plant-based with bone broth and occasional high-quality meats. Initially he juiced, for about 1 year, then switched to smoothies and included the whole plant, not just the juice. He has added several supplements to his diet.

A.J. believes his inquisitive mind has helped him on his road to recovery. Initially it was all doom and gloom, and depressing, but PQ was uplifting and explained how nutrition is powerful in healing the body. A.J. continues to monitor his blood work, and continues to dig to find the underlying cause when blood work is a little off. Today he is in remission.

For more information about healthy pleasures go to GettingHealthier.com.

ENDNOTES

[2] https://www.amazon.com/Biological-Foundations-Annals-Academy-Sciences/dp/1573313076

[3] https://www.youtube.com/watch?v=oeQfRtiY-ZM

[4] https://www.40yearsofzen.com/

[5] https://www.ncbi.nlm.nih.gov/pmc/articles/PMC1011199/

[6] https://onlinelibrary.wiley.com/doi/abs/10.1002/ijc.2910440511

[7] https://www.ncbi.nlm.nih.gov/pubmed/16549493

KEY 4
ATTITUDE/THE MIND

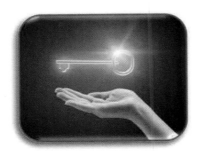

Chapter 4.2
Inspiration from Geniuses

<u>*FROM NATURE'S PHARMACY: Cinnamon*</u>

Columbus set sail over the mysterious edge of the ocean in search of spices to cover the smell of decaying food. Until refrigerators were made widely available in 1916 by General Electric, all food had a very short shelf life. Once you picked the plant or killed the animal, the process of decomposition and the rotting smell marched by quickly. The spices of the Orient, such as black pepper, turmeric, cinnamon, red peppers, ginger; were greatly prized throughout the world for making food taste and smell better. Only a few bright people had observed that these spices also made the user a bit healthier. Cinnamon is a case in point. Throughout history, cinnamon was a favorite spice mixed with sweets. Grandmas for centuries have made cinnamon apple pie for dessert. Now scientists find that cinnamon can help to lower blood glucose rises. Cinnamon used regularly as a spice in the diet can make appreciable reductions in blood glucose levels.[1]

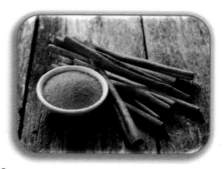

There have been many great leaders and teachers throughout human history. Following are just a few of the geniuses who inspired me. Far from an exhaustive list of global mentors, this chapter is designed to inspire, motivate, nourish, energize, and enlighten you. There is healing in this chapter. I stand on the shoulders of giants. Below listed are a few of them.

Ruth Stout (1884-1980)

Best known for her "no work" gardening books,[2] Ruth was asked about her robust mental and physical health at age 94. She told a story that changed my life. When Ruth was a 5 year old girl, her dog died. Ruth was standing in the living room, looking out the window on a rainy day while her father was burying her dog. Ruth was crying. Ruth's grandfather took Ruth gently by the shoulders and led her to the other side of the house where a rose bush was in bloom. "You were just looking out the wrong window," said her grandfather.

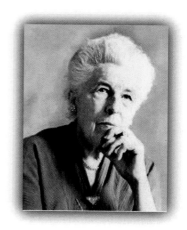

Think about it. In everyone's life, there will always be "dogs dying", or bad things happening. We have the option of looking out the window at the blooming rose bush or the burial of your favorite dog. Not talking about escapism or lacking contact with reality. We are talking about "where is your focus?" You can choose to focus on the beauty and accomplishments in life, or the failures and ugliness. It's your choice. The only real freedom and control that we have is controlling our thoughts.

Louise Hay (1926-2017).

Born into a poor and abusive home life, followed by rape and other draining experiences, Louise was diagnosed with terminal cervical cancer. Louise turned to the Church of Religious Science, reasoning that she needed to change her internal environment in order to change her external physical malady. Her book, YOU CAN HEAL YOUR LIFE, sold over 50 million copies in 30 languages. Her publishing house, Hay House, published books from over 130 authors, mostly in the health and new age field. Her compilation, GRATITUDE: A WAY OF 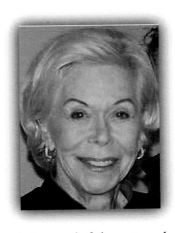 LIFE, was a game changer for me. Louise took her painful past and turned it into a sermon for millions of followers who found peace and health in her words. You must love yourself unconditionally. "You cannot be grateful and unhappy at the same time." Think about it.

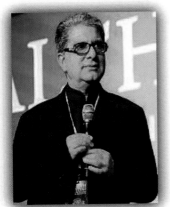

Deepak Chopra, MD (b.1946)

Chopra studied medicine in India, then residency in the US, culminating as chief of staff at New England Memorial Hospital. Chopra became involved in the meditation movement, Ayurvedic medicine from his native India, and quantum mechanics; which makes an interesting hybrid of philosophies. Dr. Chopra has written 80 books, of which 21 were on the New York Times bestseller list, and translated into 40 languages. Am impressed when someone who speaks English as a second or third language, such as Chopra, is far more articulate than those of us who were raised on English. Chopra is an artist with the spoken and written word. The science of psycho (mind) neuro (neurological system) immunology (immune system) is in its infancy. The websites that are "sanitized" by the pharmaceutical industry criticize Chopra for his abandonment of Western medicine. Yet, there are hundreds of scientific papers that support the sound bite from Dr. Chopra "Every cell in your body is eavesdropping on your thoughts."

Ignas Semmelweis, MD (1818-1865)

Semmelweis was a physician in Vienna, Austria in the 1860s when puerperal fever, or maternal fever was rampant and often lethal. Doctors would move from autopsy to the stable to deliver a horse then to the maternity ward to deliver an infant. These unsanitary conditions created nearly a 90% infection rate, roughly triple the infection rate of midwife clinics at the time. Semmelweis developed the technique of washing hands with a dilute solution of chlorine bleach. End of the problem. He could 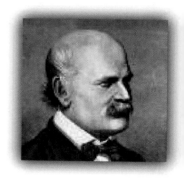 prove it. The method cost nearly nothing. No side effects.

Dr. Semmelweis's colleagues questioned him: "What is causing this problem?" Semmelweis said "I don't know." "Is it spooks?" his critics chided. Semmelweis was laughed out of the medical profession after publishing his book on his work ETIOLOGY, CONCEPT, AND PROPHYLAXIS OF CHILDBED FEVER. He died shortly after that in an asylum after being beaten by guards. Semmelweis is considered the "savior of mothers" and the pioneer of antiseptic procedures.

His technique was logical, provable, cheap, non-toxic, and extremely effective…just like using nutrition in cancer treatment. White willow bark was used for 2400 years for pain and fever. Not until 1859 was the active ingredient salicylic acid synthesized and finally the Nobel

Prize in Medicine was awarded Robert John Vane in 1982 for explaining HOW aspirin works in prostaglandin metabolism. Semmelweis saved countless lives with 3 simple words: "Wash your hands." Semmelweis was brilliant, persistent and creative in seeking a solution to a long-standing problem. Semmelweis was not the first or last doctor to be ostracized by the medical community for his pioneering methods. We need to respect people who develop effective techniques, even if we cannot explain them. There is a Semmelweis Society International charged with furthering the spirit of Dr. Semmelweis. The Semmelweis Reflex is the tendency to reject new knowledge because it contradicts established norms. We all salute Dr. Semmelweis for his brilliance and courage against an establishment that rejected a safe, cheap, effective, non-toxic solution to a serious problem. Nutrition in cancer treatment falls into the same categories. Here are three simple words to save countless lives of cancer patients: "Nourish your body."

Galileo Galilei (1564-1642)

Astronomer, physicist, and mathematician, Galileo could prove with his telescope that the earth orbited around the sun, not the other way around. At a time when the theories of Copernicus conflicted with the reigning dogma of the Catholic Church, Galileo was tried in 1615 by the Roman Inquisition and found guilty of heresy, then placed under house arrest until his death. Galileo was brilliant, inventive, creative, could prove his statements, and undeterred by opposition...just like many pioneers who have shown the value of nutrition support in cancer treatment.

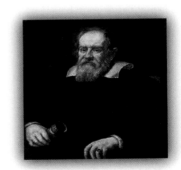

Max Gerson, MD (1881-1959)

Dr. Gerson was a German trained physician who first recognized the value of nutrition in cancer treatment. Dr. Gerson trained in Europe where food, herbs, and natural remedies were part of "standard of care". Gerson used his modified vegetarian diet to cure many people of tuberculosis when it was a primary cause of death in advanced societies.

Gerson cured Nobel Prize winner Dr. Albert Schweitzer's wife of tuberculosis, then cured Dr. Schweitzer of type 2 diabetes.

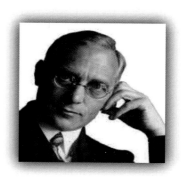

Gerson was using nutrition to cure cancer patients when the American Cancer Society (founded in 1913) insisted that nutrition had nothing to do with either the prevention or treatment of cancer. When the ACS finally issued their dietary recommendations for preventing cancer, they looked an awful lot like Dr. Gerson's diet: plant based, fresh fruit and vegetable juices, less or no meat, less sugar, less salt and more potassium. The ACS now recognizes [3] poor diet as a primary cause of cancer.

A 1994 study comparing SEER (surveillance, epidemiology and end result…aka what do we expect will happen with this patient based on the thousands who have come before him/her) with the Gerson therapy for melanoma, a poor prognostic cancer once metastasized. The Gerson program was superior in outcome for all 3 stages of melanoma examined. Gerson was chased out of the US and started his clinic in Mexico. While the Gerson program is still evolving, it took a bright mind to notice the link between nutrition and cancer and a courageous soul to battle the cancer establishment for the rest of his life.

Weston Price, DDS (1870-1948)

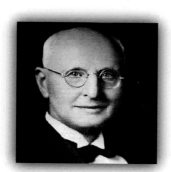

Dr. Price was a dentist who began his practice in the early part of the 20th century in Cleveland, OH. As time marched on, Dr. Price noticed the dramatic decline in the dental health of his patients. Dr. Price wondered if the huge changes in diet occurring about that time, from fresh food to refined sugar and flour, played a role in deteriorating dental health. Price and his wife, a nurse, climbed aboard the old Pan Am clippers and traveled the world visiting 12 cultures on 5 continents, taking 15,000 photographs and making copious notes.

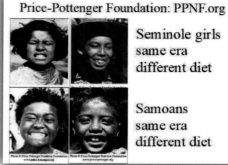

Price-Pottenger Foundation: PPNF.org

Seminole girls
same era
different diet

Samoans
same era
different diet

Price had the advantage of visiting cultures that were just beginning to embrace refined foods...he was right on the "cusp" of earthquake changes in the diet of our planet. Some people in the village ate like their ancestors and some people ate processed foods. The distinctions were blatant. People eating their native indigenous diet had wider faces which allowed for plenty of room for wisdom teeth. Dental caries were rare or non-existent in people eating native foods. Mental health and overall physical health was superior in those who ate native foods. Just like any exotic zoo animal, humans need to eat our native indigenous diet in order to have good health. The Standard American Diet (SAD) has deviated so far from our ancestral diet as to be laughable...and unhealthy. Dr.Price's work is considered a classic in modern nutrition. Many people have provocative questions on their mind. Very few of us have the time, energy, courage, intellect, and money to answer those questions. We salute Dr. Price and his wife.

Bruce Lipton, PhD (b. 1944-)

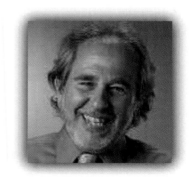

Dr. Lipton began his career in 1973 as a cell biologist teaching at medical schools. His work in stem cells earned him national recognition. He found that drugs affect not only the intended tissue, but all cells in the body, and only because we internally produce some version of every drug in the known pharmacy. Why not use the power of the mind to generate what we need rather than relying on dangerous and expensive prescription medications?

In 1982, Dr. Lipton began researching the cell membrane, which he found to be quite complex and, literally, like a computer chip. While the existing theories of health and medicine put all the control in the human gene, Dr. Lipton found that chemicals produced by our brain can radically alter the functions of the cell through a complex interplay between the substance, the cell membrane receptors, and the way the internal cell reacts to this stimuli. Dr. Lipton's groundbreaking book, <u>THE BIOLOGY OF BELIEF</u> is considered one of the founders of the vast new field of epigenetics. "Unleashing the power of consciousness, matter, and miracles" is the quest of this intellectual pioneer who has been featured throughout the media and is a highly sought after keynote speaker.

Jesus the Christ (4 BC-30 AD)

There are 2 billion Christian followers of Jesus the Anointed One. I was raised a Catholic, studied Baltimore Catechism and was an altar boy for 10 years. Completed two years at the University of Notre Dame, where I took a Bible class. Jesus was a Jewish Rabbi and entered his ministry in a time when memorizing rules and getting even with your foes was considered the status quo. Jesus offered two central rules: love God, love your neighbor as yourself. "The Kingdom of heaven is within." These brilliant sound bites baffled many of the primitive followers in those days. Today it makes perfectly good sense.

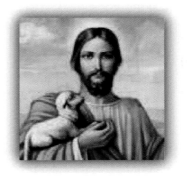

Happiness and joy are internal qualities that can be generated any time any place. Many a Hollywood or Nashville celebrity has overdosed on drugs when they had every possible physical reason to be happy: beauty, wealth, youth, fame, talent, travel, sycophants, etc. Jesus taught us to pursue peace, joy, love, happiness, kindness, forgiveness, generosity, patience, and self love. Good advice no matter your religious or spiritual persuasion. Joy is mentioned 214 times in the Bible with ¼ of those in Psalms. While understanding the plot line of life can be troubling, it is clear that there is a majestic Creator who created the universe. Try developing awe and reverence for all of life. These internal tools will help give your body, mind, and spirit the supportive environment to heal.

For more information about inspiration from geniuses go to GettingHealthier.com

---

PATIENT PROFILE

RJ was a successful attorney who was dying of stomach cancer. His doctors back home did their best with surgery, chemo and radiation. RJ came to our hospital as a stage four patient, probably going to die soon. Our psycho-neuroimmunology team found that RJ went into law because his father was a lawyer and insisted on this career path for RJ. RJ said that when he went to his law office he got a "pit in my stomach". Our psychologists worked with RJ on a new direction in life. His stomach cancer went into remission. A year later, RJ decided that he liked the money from the legal profession and went back to his law practice. His stomach cancer returned and he died soon thereafter. Stress can kill. And the mind can be an intimate partner in your recovery from cancer if you use your mind properly.

ENDNOTES

[1] Anderson, RA, Proc Nutr Soc. 2008 Feb;67(1):48-53
[2] https://www.amazon.com/Gardening-Without-Work-Aging-Indolent-ebook/dp/B01D06KKDW/ref=sr_1_1?crid=1E7J0AYR11YDV&keywords=ruth+stout+no+work+garden+book&qid=1556317698&s=gateway&sprefix=ruth+stout%2Caps%2C193&sr=8-1
[3] https://www.fightcancer.org/releases/poor-diet-cited-cause-cancer-first-time-dietary-guidelines-advisory-committee

KEY 5
EXERCISE

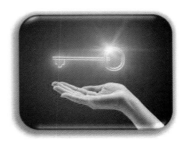

Chapter 5
Is Dis-Ease from Dis-Use of the Body?

"There is no drug in current or prospective use that holds as much promise for sustained health as a lifetime program of physical exercise."
Walter Bortz, MD, Stanford University,
<u>*Journal of American Medical Association*</u>

<u>*FROM NATURE'S PHARMACY*</u>: *Apigenin*

   Researchers at the University of California Irvine discovered a substance only found in fruits and vegetables that helps cells to die when their time has come. Programmed cell death, or apoptosis, is an intense area of research in cancer, because cancer cells "forget" to die. It is this loss of apoptosis that makes cancer such a difficult disease to treat and usually creates chemo resistance, so that even if the chemo was working in the beginning, it stops working due to this cellular glitch in cancer cells. Apigenin is a substance found in fresh red and green fruits and vegetables that causes p53 to make cancer cells die and even increases the kill rate when cancer cells are given chemo. This study was funded by the National Institutes of Health and published in Proceedings of the National Academy of Sciences.[1] We have known for centuries that a diet rich in fruits and vegetables was protective against cancer and many other diseases. With modern science we are beginning to understand "why" this works.

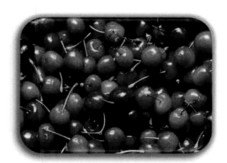

While 40% of Americans will develop cancer in their lifetime, you can cut that number in half simply by exercising 3 times each week. Exercise in animals with tumors produced a 60% reduction in tumor incidence and growth. Ballroom dancing at least once per week lowers the risk of Alzheimer's disease by 73%. Exercise may tie with meditation when it comes to the simplest, cheapest, most effective way of improving your health.

Original Investigation [FREE]

June 2016

Association of Leisure-Time Physical Activity With Risk of 26 Types of Cancer in 1.44 Million Adults

Steven C. Moore, PhD, MPH[1]; I-Min Lee, MBBS, ScD[2]; Elisabete Weiderpass, PhD[3,4,5,6]; et al

> Author Affiliations | Article Information

JAMA Intern Med. 2016;176(6):816-825. doi:10.1001/jamainternmed.2016.1548

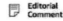 Editorial
Comment

Exercise Improves Survival Rate of Cancer Patients

A 2013 research study involving mice, found that mice that exercised on a treadmill for one hour daily for five days a week over a period of 32 weeks had a significantly lower risk of liver cancer compared to their sedentary counterparts.

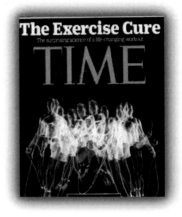

Another study indicates that shedding a mere 5 percent of body weight increases survival rate of breast cancer patients by 20 percent. And yet another study at Yale University, involving 5000 people with breast cancer, found that three hours of brisk walking per week reduced mortality rate by 46 percent. Many other studies have come up with similar findings. And yet, even without these cancer-focused studies, it is well known that regular physical exercise helps keep the body healthy. It sharpens the mind, reduces stress, and helps you sleep better.

In a groundbreaking study published in 2016, researchers found that exercise in tumor bearing mice reduced tumor burden:[2]

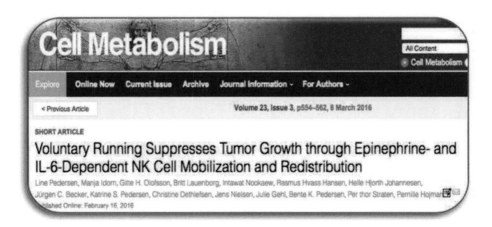

"...a 60% reduction in tumor incidence and growth across five different tumor models...induced upregulation of pathways associated with immune function and Natural Killer cell infiltration...Together these results link exercise, epinephrine, and IL-6 to NK mobilization and redistribution and, ultimately, to control of tumor growth."

If any cancer drug could reduce tumor incidence and growth by 60% it would be international headlines. Yet you cannot patent or even sell exercise. Exercise could be a crucial key in your cancer recovery.

How Does Exercise Improve Health?

Health benefits of exercise are not limited to certain conditions. When cancer patients and cancer survivors exercise regularly, they set themselves up for the following health benefits:

- Reduction of stress, anxiety and risk of depression
- Enhanced detoxification
- "cooking" cancer and infectious cells through elevated temperature
- Increased production of endorphins; feel-good hormones associated with fighting disease
- Improved flow of lymph fluids which strengthens the immune system
- Better quality and quantity of sleep
- Prevention of constipation
- Higher energy levels
- Reduced fatigue
- Improved heart health
- Better blood circulation
- Lower risk of blood clots
- Improved appetite
- Stronger, healthier bones
- Healthy weight management
- Improved balance and posture
- Reduced dependence on others
- Better self-esteem and self-worth
- Increased musculoskeletal strength

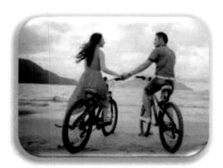

- Better quality of life
- Reduced nausea

How to Exercise During and After Treatment

Physical exercise helps during and after cancer treatment. Some therapists advise patients to start exercising as soon as possible following cancer diagnosis and commencement of treatment.

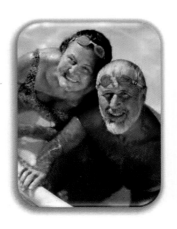

Your ability and intensity depends on whether or not you were physically active prior to the diagnosis. If you have been exercising hard, you may need to slow down a bit. Those who begin exercising during or following treatment, need to start with gentle exercises and to build up the intensity and duration of exercise as your body adjusts. As you commence exercise to help in your recuperation, it helps to consult your doctor and a physical therapist for any suggestions and guidance.

This is even more important for elderly persons and those suffering, or with a risk of suffering from conditions such as heart disease, osteoporosis and arthritis.

How Much Exercise Should You Do?

The idea of exercising is to keep your body fit. To achieve this, you need to indulge in regular physical activity. More than 20 studies have found that the risk of cancer recurrence is lower for survivors who maintain a physically active lifestyle. These studies have been carried out on people with different cancers, including ovarian, prostate, breast and colorectal.

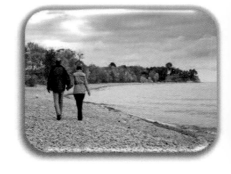

The American Cancer Society says that cancer survivors benefit more by doing the following:

- Exercising regularly
- Exercising for 2 ½ hours or more per week
- Adopting challenging strength training as part of the exercise program for two days or more per week

Types of Exercise to Slow Down Cancer

There are many types of exercise to choose from including the following:

- Riding a bicycle
- Yoga
- Swimming
- Ballroom (with a partner) dancing, shown to reduce the risk of Alzheimer's by 73%
- Walking
- Gardening
- Cleaning your car
- Weightless workout: pushups, chin ups, sit ups, dips, squats
- Stationary bike riding
- Pilates or Total Gym, resistance training using body weight
- Climbing stairs
- Mowing your lawn
- Wearing a pedometer helps you track your physical activity level so that you can steadily increase it

How to Exercise to Aid Recovery from Cancer

Here's how you can maintain a regular exercise routine:

- Decide what exercises you will be doing
- Draw up a routine
- Exercise regularly
- Exercise outdoors when possible so you enjoy the fresh air

- Include resting intervals in your exercise routine
- Drink 8 glasses of water or more per day
- Choose exercises that you enjoy doing
- Set goals – short-term and long-term
- Vary your exercise types
- Keep track of your exercises using a pedometer or a chart

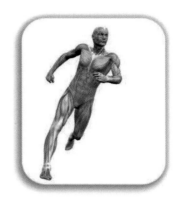

- Ask your doctor for pain control medications when necessary
- Reward yourself when you reach exercise targets
- Ask for help when you need it
- Enlist your friends in your exercises

Avoid Exercise In Case Of The Following:

- Anemia
- Low white blood cell count
- If you have mineral (electrolyte) imbalance especially due to vomiting and diarrhea
- If you have pain, nausea or vomiting
- Avoid water exercises in case you have an inserted feeding tube or catheter
- Avoid exposure to the sun if undergoing radiation
- Avoid extreme exercises during treatment and immediately after treatment
- Consult your doctor in case of injury, sudden weight gain, swelling, bleeding, shortness of breath after minimal exercise or similar

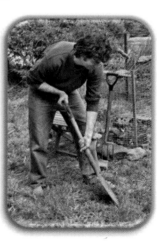

For more information about how exercise can benefit you go to GettingHealthier.com.

PATIENT PROFILE

K.B. was diagnosed with thyroid cancer in 2014. Her consultation with PQ was August 2015. Prior to diagnosis her diet consisted of low-quality burgers, sodas and sugary foods. K.B. made significant changes to her diet and improved her nutrition and now exercises regularly. K.B has undertaken many natural therapies and believes the immunotherapy (from South America) was very helpful in her recovery. K.B. also takes many supplements daily including fish oil, turmeric, iodine, beta glucan, iv's including with glutathione and vitamin C. K.B. also makes juices, smoothies and plant-based protein drinks almost daily. Today K.B. is in complete remission and feels great.

ENDNOTES

[1] Cai X, et al "Inhibition of Thr55 phosphorylation restores p53 nuclear localization and sensitizes cancer cells to DNA damage" PNAS 2008; DOI: 10.1073/pnas.0804608105.
[2] https://www.ncbi.nlm.nih.gov/pubmed/?term=voluntary+running+suppresses+tumor+growth

KEY 6
Detoxification

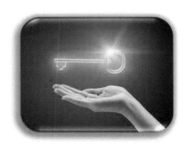

Chapter 6
Cleanse Your Body

"We've got to do something about our pollution issue. My kid's water pistol gets jammed." Unknown

FROM NATURE'S PHARMACY: *Green Tea*

Green tea may be the <u>healthiest beverage on earth</u>.[1] About 30% of the dry weight of green tea is polyphenols, including EGCG, which has powerful health giving effects in the human body. Green tea has been shown to reduce inflammation, lower cancer risk, lower heart disease risk, slow down cancer growth, improve

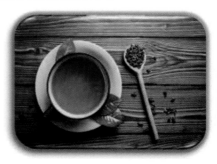

weight loss, powerful antioxidant, anti-aging, improves brain function, <u>reduces anxiety</u>.[2] Buy organic green tea. Make green sun tea. Drink often. Capsules of green tea might even be a good idea for turbo-charging your health. Cheap, no prescription, time tested for millennia, vast array of health benefits. What are you waiting for?

Of the <u>10 million tons</u> [3] of toxic substances released annually by industry around the world, 2 million tons are probable carcinogens. Of the <u>80,000 chemicals</u> [4] in use in the USA, 60,000 were released without any data on safety in humans. The burden of proof rests on society to prove something is hazardous. Not easy to do when you realize that asbestos was approved by the Environmental Protection Agency, because they could not prove that asbestos was toxic. Asbestos has been banned in most developed countries, but still used in many developing countries and <u>now kills at least 255,000 people</u> [5] each year around the world.

43% of Americans breathe air that is unsafe, according to the American lung association. We add 1 billion pounds of pesticides to our food crops annually. Of the 3000 food additives in the American food supply, FDA has no knowledge of at least 1000 of these, due to loopholes in the law via "generally regarded as safe" or GRAS status. 70% of Americans drink tap water that, by law, must contain fluoride, <u>a known poison</u>.[6]

And we haven't even started on the issue of synergism. With toxins, 1 + 1 might equal 500 or more. <u>Professor Ershoff in 1976</u> fed rats a low fiber diet along with various combinations of FDA approved food additives: 2% of diet sodium cyclamate, and/or FD&C red dye #2, and/or polyoxyethylene sorbitan monostearate. Group 1, 2 and 3 of the rats were fed only one of the above additives. Results were unremarkable. Group 4 was fed sodium cyclamate with red dye #2. The results were weight loss, hair loss, and diarrhea. Group 5 was fed all 3 food additives with the results being extensive weight loss, then death of all animals by day 14. Very few of the

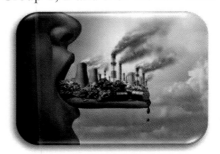

chemicals that we are exposed to have been tested for safety. NONE of the chemicals are tested in combination, as above. And we wonder why we have a cancer epidemic on our hands.

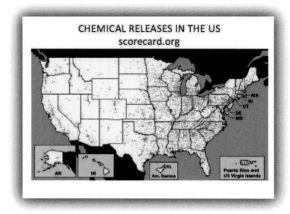

The American Cancer Society and American Medical Association agree that toxins are a main cause of many illnesses in western society, from Parkinson's, to cancer, to birth defects, autoimmune diseases, and more. In order to heal, you need to address the issue of the toxins that surround us, how to avoid them, and how to eliminate the toxins in your body.

The Environmental Working Group conducted a study [7] examining the placental blood of 10 newborn babies randomly chosen from a Red Cross national cord blood collection program…not because the mothers worked near any chemicals. Of the 287 different chemicals detected in the newborn's cord blood, 180 cause cancer and 217 cause nervous system

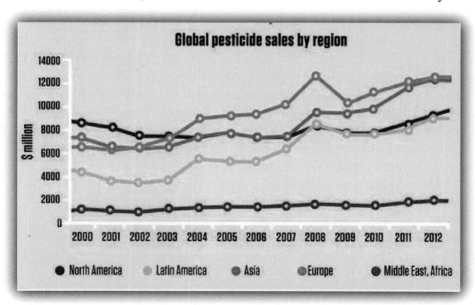

problems. Included in this hit parade of poisons was pesticides, mercury, Teflon, Scotchgard, and wastes from coal, gasoline, and garbage. In newborns. Imagine what is in your body, unless you make a concerted effort to limit your intake of toxins and make a heroic effort at eliminating the toxins already in your body.

There is a Great Pacific Garbage Patch with at least 80,000 tons of discarded plastic covering an area of 620,000 square miles, or twice the size of Texas in the middle of the Pacific Ocean. Plastic has found its way into the food chain of fish. By 2050 there will be more plastic in the ocean than fish. We need to do something. Quickly.

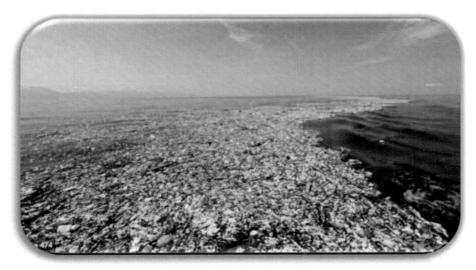

Brain tumors are the leading cause of death among childhood cancers. Nothing is more gut wrenching than watching a bald child on TV soliciting donations for the hospital. Meanwhile, researchers studied 540 children with brain cancer and found that the more processed meats (bacon, sausage, salami, bologna) with nitrosamides mother ate while pregnant, the higher the risk for brain tumor in the child. Taking prenatal supplements lowered, but did not eliminate, the brain cancer risk when eating processed meat.[8]

Glyphosate (Roundup) is an herbicide first patented [9] in 1964 to clean boiler pipes. Glyphosate was patented again in 1974 as an herbicide, then again in 2003 as an antibiotic. The World Health Organization has listed glyphosate as a "probable carcinogen", which was instrumental in a jury awarding a patient with non-Hodgkins lymphoma $289 verdict against Monsanto, the manufacturer. A couple was recently awarded $2 billion for the cancer they contracted from Roundup use. There are over 12,000 cases pending against Bayer/Monsanto for Roundup-induced cancer. 95 million pounds of glyphosate are used annually in the US.

Old Fashioned Toxins

Around 1890, John Snow [10] was a scientist in London who identified the massive cholera outbreak in the city as being caused by human feces contamination in the drinking water. Snow had to overcome unthinkable barriers to convince scientists and government officials of the cause and solution to this epidemic that killed 52,000 people. Thomas Crapper made toilets widely available in London around that time, and cholera epidemics have virtually disappeared where toilets are used. Cholera killed about 40 million people in India [11] in the 19th century.

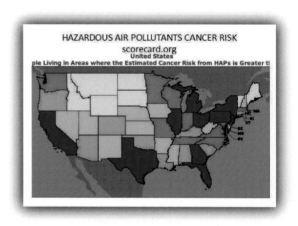

Mercury is a metal that is liquid at room temperature and does not rust, making it the perfect ingredient for dental fillings. Until you realize that mercury is the most toxic non-radioactive substance on earth.

Humans have zero tolerance for mercury in the body. Mercury causes [12] neurological problems, autoimmune diseases, possibly autism, and probably cancer. Mercury was commonly used in dental fillings throughout the 1800s. In 1926 a prominent German scientist [13] Alfred Stock found that mercury fillings were the cause of his health problems.

Stock campaigned to have mercury removed from amalgam formulas, to no avail. Mercury is still used throughout most of the world in fillings and as a preservative in vaccines.

Lead was a known poison [14] when it was first discovered in 1854. Throughout most of the early 20th century, lead was used liberally in paints and as an anti-knock compound in car gasoline, generating millions of tons of lead in the air. Not until decades of evidence was gathered showing that lead causes developmental problems in children, and heart disease and cancer in adults, was lead finally banned from gasoline in 1975.

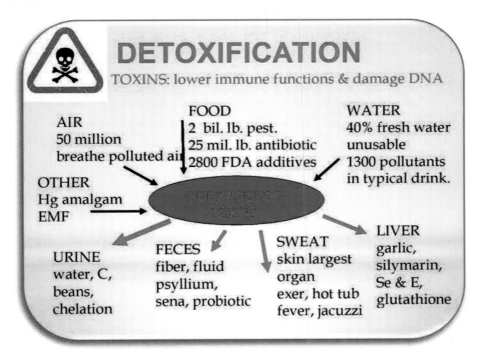

Government in Action or Government Inaction?

And if you think the Environmental Protection Agency is protecting the public, think again. E.G. Vallianatos was a high ranking official at the EPA for 25 years and upon retirement wrote a scathing book, POISON SPRING, [15] about the EPA being run by the chemical industry it is supposed to regulate. Industry released 60,000 different chemicals upon American consumers with no safety data. Most lipstick contains lead, a potent toxin. And on its goes.

Cigarette smoking has been called the deadliest artifact ever invented, with 1.5 million deaths per year [16] from lung cancer alone. Cigarettes were known to be dangerous in the 19th century, but are still legal everywhere in the world. These are just a few isolated examples of where toxins were known to be toxic for decades before they could be removed from circulation or are still allowed. The rise in cancer parallels our indiscreet use of chemicals, electromagnetic fields, and radiation. To make all this more illogical, chemotherapy and radiation that are used to treat cancer, also cause cancer. [17]

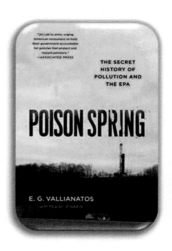

Toxins could be categorized as:
1) Volatile organic chemicals, from industry and agriculture
2) Tobacco
3) Drugs, prescription and recreation
4) Fungal by products, e.g. aflatoxin
5) Heavy metals, including mercury, lead, cadmium, arsenic, aluminum and other metals
6) Auto-intoxication, as by products from our gut, especially for those with an imbalance in gut microbiome
7) Electromagnetic fields, cell phone towers, WiFi, high voltage power lines, radar, etc.
8) Radiation, X-rays, radioactive fallout, sunlight, etc.

Toxins are known to affect many parameters of the human body, from immune suppression, to hormone disruptors, to DNA mutagens, and more.

To beat cancer, you must initiate a serious detoxification program. Let's keep this simple. Here are my recommendations:
1) Eat organic. If you eat commercial produce that does not have a peeling (grapes, spinach), then soak the food before consuming it.

2) Drink lots of purified water. Buy a water purifier for your kitchen tap and use stainless steel or glass drinking bottles.

3) Make sure that you eat enough fiber to have daily bowel movements.

4) Use simple products. Glass, stainless steel. Avoid Teflon and aluminum cooking utensils. Use simple soaps, cosmetics and anything that comes in contact with your body. Question any expensive or unnecessary substance being applied to your body. For example, 61% of lipsticks tested contained lead.[18] Use clean, simple, natural products.

5) Replace mercury fillings with non-mercury amalgams.

6) Avoid areas of high voltage. Use the speakerphone or ear buds feature on your cell phone. Use an EMF meter [19] to learn about hot spots in your home and workplace.

7) Use a sauna or far infrared sauna [20] to sweat and detoxify your body.

8) Take detox supplements that help to clean the liver, such as cilantro and silymarin.

9) Do what you can to clean up your corner of the world. We need to improve our stewardship of this garden planet we are fortunate to occupy. Good planets are hard to come by.

For more information about detoxification go to GettingHealthier.com.

PATIENT PROFILE
GP was diagnosed with uterine cancer. She had been healthy all her life. A non-smoker, non-drinker and rarely gets sick. Her consultation with PQ was March 14, 2016. Following her consultation with PQ, GP improved her diet, adding more plant-based foods and cut out sugar. She also makes a point of exercising daily, which she contributes to her current good health. GP took many nutrition supplements for about 18 months. GP is currently in remission (2 years) and feels very good.

ENDNOTES

[1] https://www.ncbi.nlm.nih.gov/pubmed/28864169

[2] https://www.ncbi.nlm.nih.gov/pubmed/18296328

[3] http://www.worldometers.info/view/toxchem/

[4] https://www.pbs.org/newshour/science/it-could-take-centuries-for-epa-to-test-all-the-unregulated-chemicals-under-a-new-landmark-bill

[5] https://en.wikipedia.org/wiki/Asbestos

[6] https://articles.mercola.com/sites/articles/archive/2012/05/21/fluoride-health-hazards.aspx

[7] https://www.ewg.org/research/body-burden-pollution-newborns

[8] https://cebp.aacrjournals.org/content/5/8/599.short

[9] https://gmofreeusa.org/research/glyphosate/glyphosate-overview/

[10] https://books.google.com/books?hl=en&lr=&id=l1Zer0QT4tgC&oi=fnd&pg=PR7&dq=toxic+environmental+exposures&ots=J7fpLi4ufg&sig=YndooAuWBl99GpneP05LCoMz8Yw#v=onepage&q=toxic%20environmental%20exposures&f=false

[11] https://en.wikipedia.org/wiki/Cholera_outbreaks_and_pandemics

[12] https://iaomt.org/resources/dental-mercury-facts/amalgam-fillings-danger-human-health/

[13] https://dentistinnewhavenct.com/a-history-of-amalgam-fillings/

[14] https://www.smithsonianmag.com/smart-news/leaded-gas-poison-invented-180961368/

[15] https://www.amazon.com/dp/B00IAMKD4S/ref=dp-kindle-redirect?_encoding=UTF8&btkr=1

[16] https://tobaccocontrol.bmj.com/content/21/2/87

[17] http://www.greenmedinfo.com/blog/does-chemo-radiation-actually-make-cancer-more-malignant

[18] http://www.safecosmetics.org/get-the-facts/regulations/us-laws/lead-in-lipstick/

[19] https://www.amazon.com/KKmeter-Electromagnetic-Radiation-Detector-Handheld/dp/B07B9WHGN3/ref=asc_df_B07B9WHGN3/?tag=hyprod-20&linkCode=df0&hvadid=312096362814&hvpos=1o1&hvnetw=g&hvrand=12843748391170450523&hvpone=&hvptwo=&hvqmt=&hvdev=c&hvdvcmdl=&hvlocint=&hvlocphy=9031288&hvtargid=aud-643574997066:pla-511755129834&psc=1

[20] https://www.amazon.com/SereneLife-Portable-Infrared-Person-Weight/dp/B0711XW4P3/ref=sr_1_3?crid=1N6MFDXAGD84M&keywords=far+infrared+sauna&qid=1555711211&s=gateway&sprefix=far+infra+red%2Cindustrial%2C196&sr=8-3

KEY 7
ENERGY ALIGNMENT

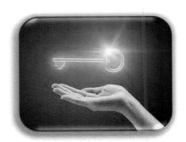

Chapter 7
Bolstering the Human Power Grid

"I sing the body electric."
Walt Whitman

FROM NATURE'S PHARMACY: Avocados

10,000 years ago, natives of central Mexico were eating avocados, which are technically a fruit, not unlike a green cherry with a large pit in the middle. Mexico still produces 1/3 of the world's avocados. <u>Avocados are a rich source</u> of potassium (more than a banana), vitamins K, B-6, C, folate, pantothenic acid, E; and a fantastic source of monounsaturated fats that are heart healthy. 77% of the 160 kcal in your average avocado comes from oleic acid, which is the fat that made olive oil so healthy.

People who eat avocados regularly are less likely to be overweight and half as likely to have metabolic syndrome, a condition that often leads to heart disease. Avocados reduce inflammation, help us to absorb antioxidants found in other plant foods, have anti-cancer capabilities, carry a rich supply of fiber, and much more. Slice avocados on your next salad or make guacamole from mashed avocado with salsa and lemon juice. Healthy pleasures at their best.

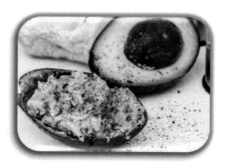

If your heart stops, a doctor may use a defibrillator to pump 200-1700 volts into your heart to get it started again. Electro convulsive therapy involves pumping 180-460 volts into the brain of a patient to treat depression or other severe conditions. Compare those numbers to the 110 volts in your home electric outlets. The human body contains somewhere between 7 and 114 chakras, or energy centers.

A human body at rest generates about 100 watts of power, or enough to light up 10 LED bulbs in your home. The human body is a maze and a complex network of energy pathways. Each of your cells generates around -20 to -25 mvolts. Healing requires a higher voltage, closer to -50 mvolts. If power is flowing optimally, then health is the result. If power is disrupted, then sickness is the consequence.

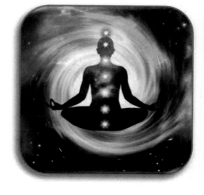

This field of energy medicine has the potential to provide extraordinary healing and restorative capacity to humans, yet is not considered "standard of care" by the medical establishment and is openly discouraged.

Nikola Tesla (1856-1943) was one of the most creative geniuses of the 19th and 20th centuries. Tesla proposed means by which energy (light, electricity) could heal and energize humans. Jerry Tennant, MD cured himself of a debilitating brain condition using electricity and came to the conclusion **HEALING IS VOLTAGE.**[1] Dr. Tennant developed a BioModulator to help establish a healthier current in the body. Due to the severe restrictions of modern medicine, Dr. Tennant can only offer these energy therapies to people under the umbrella as a pastoral health practitioner.

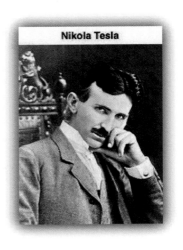

Nikola Tesla

Dr. Reinard Voll in Germany in 1952 developed a fascinating electro acupuncture device for healing, electro acupuncture according to Voll, or EAV.[2] Royal Rife (1888-1971) developed a device that purportedly could inflict a selectively lethal vibration on cancer cells without harming the patient. Pulsed electromagnetic field (PEMF) is a relatively new therapy that may recharge the body from something similar to the earth's magnetic field. The American Cancer Society and American Medical Association have staunchly placed these electrical treatments in the "quack" category. Meanwhile, talented clinicians are busy developing electromagnetic fields that can heal, as explained in their peer reviewed science journal article:[3] "Targeted treatment of cancer with radiofrequency electromagnetic fields."

Frequencies

All of the universe vibrates. Some vibrations or frequencies can be seen, some heard, most neither. Physicists are quick to explain the role of vibration, frequencies, electricity, magnetic forces, electrons, electron donors (antioxidants) vs. electron thieves (free radicals), pH (acid/base) into a neat cohesive package. Doctors are quick to ignore all of this data and the potential for healing through energy.

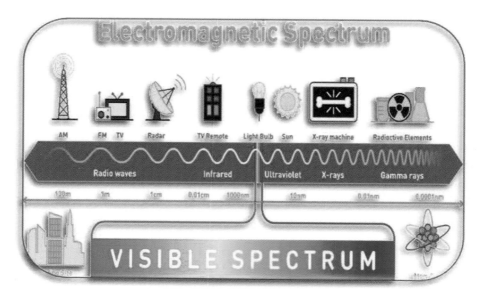

EMF Smog

There is disturbing evidence that high voltage power lines increase the risk for birth defects and cancer in young people. Cell phones plastered to the head, especially in young people with thinner skulls, can cause brain cancer. Some people are concerned about the health effects of the newly introduced 5G cell phone towers. Unless you live in a remote village, we are all bathed in electromagnetic fields, microwaves, Wi-Fi, AM, FM, cell phone towers, and industrial power grids. We are all participating, involuntarily, in a huge experiment to see if these abundant electro-magnetic fields (EMF smog) are toxic to some or most of us. There are numerous devices to measure the EMF in your home. Suggest that you buy one. There are numerous devices that offer protection from electromagnetic fields. I do not endorse nor discourage any of them. Do your own research.

Meridians and Corona

Simyan Kirlian was a Russian scientist who discovered in 1939 a unique technique to photograph the corona discharge of the human body, which can be changed based upon mood or health. This bioelectrography is used in some alternative clinics. Acupuncture and acupressure address the issue of energy, or Chi (aka Qi, pronounced "chee") by stimulating the 361 acupressure points on the human body that are arranged into 12 meridians, each relating to an organ or system in the body. Doctors of chiropractic and osteopathic medicine manipulate the human skeletal frame to encourage proper energy flow. Many massage techniques rely on improving energy flow to speed healing.

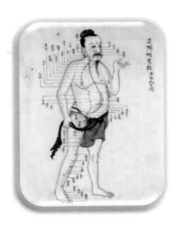

Acupuncture

A close friend, Will, was a medical student from the US sent as an ambassador to China. Will was asked to observe and photograph a brain surgery operation, in which the only anesthesia given were electrodes from a motorcycle battery connected to the patient's ear lobes. The top of the patient's skull was sawed off with the patient fully awake. Brain exposed, the patient spoke to the visiting medical students "welcome to my surgery". Will did finish his MD but could never go back to routine allopathy. Although acupuncture has been practiced since the Stone Age, the formal science of acupuncture dates back to the Ming Dynasty in 1368. The National Institutes of Health [4] even admits that acupuncture has merit in pain and symptomatic relief.

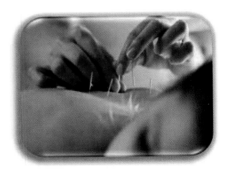

Guitar legend, Eric Clapton, was healed of a lifetime of drug and alcohol addiction using auricular (ear) electro acupuncture, and founded The Cross Roads (title of one of Eric's albums) center in the Caribbean to help others with this treatment.[5] After so many failures at drug withdrawal programs, this program was a lifesaver to Clapton.

Electricity

In the classic horror film, Dr. Frankenstein, the mad inventor sews together dead body parts to create a monster, then infuses the monster with electricity from a lightning strike, which brings the monster to life. Fiction, but not totally crazy. About 500 Americans are struck by lightning each year, with about a 10% mortality rate, or 50 deaths. Every day there are about 8 million lightning strikes around the world, each strike carrying 1 billion volts making Mother Earth a giant battery emitting electrons (antioxidants) by the trillions. Since our ancestors walked barefoot on the earth, thus being charged by earth's electricity, earth grounding has gained momentum in the scientific community [6] for zero toxicity, low cost, and great potential for healing.

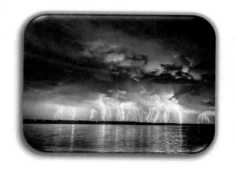

It is most intriguing that lightning can cure some severe illnesses.[7] In 1911 a 65 year old woman was cured of her lifetime deafness via a lightning strike. A woman in Oklahoma who had been wheelchair bound with multiple sclerosis was able to walk after being hit by lightning. There are many more similar bizarre cases of healing from lightning. No, I am not suggesting that you do your Benjamin Franklin impression and go out in a lightning storm with a kite and a key. Before you are through with this chapter, you will be impressed at the extraordinary energy field that is your body. Nurture your energy pathways, and healing is more likely.

Electrolyte Soup

Basic chemistry to understand life revolves around pH (potential hydrogens, or acid/base balance) and prooxidant (electron thief) vs. antioxidant (electron donor). Acid/base dictates your body's ability to absorb oxygen, which then dictates whether your cells will turn mutant and become cancerous. Your body generates electricity in elegant ways, including just like the old fashioned car battery. Your body is 2/3 water with a rich mixture of 4% body weight as dozens of minerals, of which 13 are considered essential. Those minerals create the electrolyte "soup" that allows the body to generate electricity and conduct electrical impulses along nerves that eventually fire muscles. Most western diets are deficient in magnesium, potassium, and many trace minerals, including lithium, selenium, chromium, sulfur, vanadium, boron, and more. Before the advent of light bulbs and electricity, most heat, cooking, and light came from burning wood; and the wood ashes (mostly minerals) were sprinkled back over the soil, providing a neat circle of fertilizing the soil with essential minerals. Minerals perform many essential functions in the human body, including upregulating and down regulating gene switches and providing the basis for generating electricity.

Light Therapy

Some therapists use light therapy to heal. There are over 50,000 peer reviewed articles on the therapeutic application of laser therapy, as encapsulated in the academically affiliated textbook by Harvard professor Michael Hamblin in PHOTOBIOMODULATION.[8] Since sunlight is the

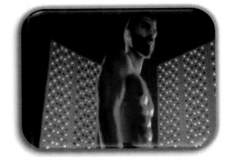

beginning of life on earth via photosynthesis, it seems obvious that there is healing potential in selective use of the light spectrum. Babies born with jaundice are exposed to a particular light therapy that induces oxidation of the bilirubin, thus curing the jaundice.

Sound Therapy

Some therapists use sound as a healing modality. Mitchell Gaynor, MD was a triple board certified oncologist working with cancer patients in NYC and employing music therapy among other modalities.[9] Dr. Gaynor died mysteriously in 2015 at the age of 59 with the alleged cause of death listed as suicide. Eileen Day McKusick has developed a healing modality involving tuning forks that interrupt or dissolve disease frequencies in her book TUNING THE HUMAN BIOFIELD.[10]

Homeopathy

Homeopathy is a form of healing developed by Samuel Hahnemann in 1796 with fundamental tenets that "like cures like" and "dilution with succussion (shaking) increases potency. Homeopathy is endorsed by the German government as a legitimate healing modality, and is used by 11% of Germans. The Royal Family in England has endorsed homeopathy for 3 generations. The Queen Mother of England was the Royal Patron of Homeopathy and lived to 101 years. Meanwhile, the FDA has considered homeopathy ineffective. Tech giants on the internet have cleansed their data bases of homeopathic remedies.

Allopathic medicine is based on concentration of active ingredients. Homeopathy takes the exact opposite approach, the more you dilute the substance, the more potent it becomes. These two sciences cannot peacefully co-exist, until you bring in the science of energy medicine. Homeopathic preparations have nothing more than the "fingerprint" of the original atom or molecule, which is why they work. Energy medicine with no toxicity.

Cultivating Chi

Tai chi is an ancient Chinese martial art, also known as shadow boxing. Tai chi can be used to gather energy into the core for healing. Qigong is a Chinese martial art and holistic system of body posture, coordinated movement, breathing, meditation, and more…all designed to cultivate Chi, or life energy. The superhuman feats of these masters leaves a Westerner 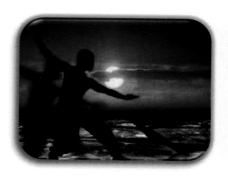 bewildered. Then we can add in the documented fields of quantum physics, once called "spooky" by Albert Einstein. Remote viewing and extra sensory perception as documented by a Stanford physicist.[11]

What to Do?

Protect yourself from unnecessary EMF exposure. If you use a microwave oven, stand at least 2 feet from the oven while operating it.

Use the speakerphone or earbuds with your cell phone. Working with your doctor, use any or all of the above-mentioned modalities to improve the life force within your body. Use an inversion board, with your doctor's permission, to allow your spinal column to stretch out and improve the flow of Chi through your body.

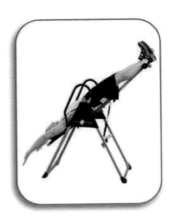

This chapter introduces the essential topic of the human body as a battery, full of energy "freeways", connected to a non-local consciousness. We need to research, measure, enhance and respect the body electric. To ignore the body electric would be unscientific and foolish. Harnessing the healing power of our electrical field is essential medicine for the 21st century. Our survival as a species and your healing as an individual are at stake.

For more information about energy alignment go to GettingHealthier.com.

PATIENT PROFILE

Multiple myeloma: a relatively rare and poor prognostic cancer in which cancer cells crowd out the healthy cells in the bone marrow

J.H. was a 41 year old white male diagnosed with multiple myeloma in 2001. JH had a consultation with PQ in which we discussed lifestyle changes, including diet and nutrition supplements. JH worked with his doctor on medical therapies for his condition. JH went into remission, was able to re-establish his pilot's license, continue to work as an attorney, and bestselling fiction author. JH had an excellent quality of life for the next 14 years, at which he went into a steep decline and died.

K.Q. was a 41 year old white male diagnosed with multiple myeloma in 1999. PQ worked with KQ to provide guidelines for lifestyle changes, including nutrition and supplements. KQ's oncologist said: "If you take any of these supplements, then I will not work with you." KQ died 18 months later.

Michael Gearin-Tosh was a white male Oxford professor who was diagnosed with multiple myeloma in 1994 at the age of 54. He was told that he would die soon without conventional therapy. MGT took a different route for his therapies, including using Beating Cancer with Nutrition, intravenous vitamin C, high dose nutrition supplements, and more. MGT went into remission and lived another 11 years before passing away in 2005. Dr. Gearin-Tosh wrote a book, LIVING PROOF, A MEDICAL MUTINY to detail his journey toward wellness for longer than anyone expected.

ENDNOTES

[1] https://www.amazon.com/Healing-Voltage-Handbook-Jerry-Tennant/dp/1453649166/ref=sr_1_1?crid=3VDS2XCAO57C1&keywords=healing+is+voltage+by+dr.+jerry+tennant&qid=1559940921&s=gateway&sprefix=jerry+tennant%2Caps%2C194&sr=8-1

[2] https://www.biontologyarizona.com/dr-reinhard-voll/

[3] https://www.ncbi.nlm.nih.gov/pmc/articles/PMC3845545/

[4] https://newsinhealth.nih.gov/2011/02/understanding-acupuncture

[5] https://crossroadsantigua.org/lp/alcohol-inpatient-treatment/

[6] https://www.ncbi.nlm.nih.gov/pmc/articles/PMC3265077/

[7] https://www.theguardian.com/news/2014/jul/27/weatherwatch-cured-by-lightning

[8] https://www.amazon.com/Low-Level-Light-Therapy-Photobiomodulation-Tutorial/dp/151061415X/ref=sr_1_1?keywords=photobiomodulation&qid=1559942106&s=books&sr=1-1

[9] https://www.amazon.com/Healing-Power-Sound-Recovery-Life-Threatening/dp/1570629552/ref=sr_1_1?keywords=mitch+gaynor&qid=1559940710&s=gateway&sr=8-1

[10] https://www.amazon.com/Tuning-Human-Biofield-Healing-Vibrational/dp/1620552469

[11] https://www.amazon.com/gp/product/B00SKF0WLY/ref=dbs_a_def_rwt_hsch_vapi_tkin_p1_i0

KEY 8
MICROBIOME

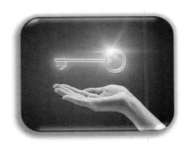

Chapter 8
Healing Begins in Your Gut

"All diseases begin in the gut."
Hippocrates, father of modern medicine, circa 370 BC

FROM NATURE'S PHARMACY: Yogurt

In 1908, Eli Metchnikoff, PhD won the Nobel Prize in Medicine for his work on discovering how immune warriors (phagocytes) gobble up invaders. At the same time, Dr. Metchnikoff advocated regular consumption of yogurt to improve the immune system via the gut.

Yogurt is fermented milk. There are many organisms that can be used as starters for yogurt, but among the more common strains of bacteria are Lactobacillus acidophilus. Yogurt contains protein and calcium in abundance. While commercial milk consumption has been linked to prostate cancer, all data on yogurt shows improvement in health. <u>Health benefits of yogurt</u> are legendary and scientifically rock solid. [1] Gut problems, including irritable bowel syndrome, diarrhea from pelvic radiation or food poisoning, often disappear with yogurt consumption. Yogurt colonizes the gut with friendly 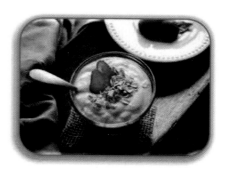 bacteria that dramatically improve our health, as you will read in this chapter. Yogurt that has been diluted with sugar is less healthy than plain yogurt with some fresh fruit added.

We have the seeds of our demise within our gut. Those same "seeds" are 100 trillion microorganisms which will become part of 21st century medicine. Throughout history, "gut shot or stabbed" meant an awful death, because the bacteria from the colon will invade the bloodstream and cause septicemia, a nasty way to go. However, if kept in their "dormitory" of the gut, these critters become an important part of healing from cancer.

"With a little help from my friends..." sang the Beatles. In the petroleum age we live, oil refineries around the world take in black thick crude oil and render it, via the catalytic cracking process, into hundreds of different chemicals that can be used in modern society, including gasoline and plastics. Child's play compared to the human gut. Humans take a carrot, peach, or fish fillet and digest it down to molecules that can slide through the digestive wall, into the bloodstream, and be usable to the body. This is no small task. The stomach produces acid that would eat a hole in your home carpet. But a healthy stomach can handle that. The intestines dump about a quart daily of digestive juices that take the necklace of your food, as polymers, and break it down to individual beads. Your digestive tract has the surface area of a tennis court.

autoimmune diseases in the 1950s and 1960s with the enthusiastic use of antibiotics. His book, THE MISSING DIAGNOSIS is still a classic[6]. Antibiotics kill all bacteria in the gut, the good and the bad, leaving yeast to thrive in the absence of competition. Yeast infections then became common, as told by William Crook, MD in THE YEAST CONNECTION.

The Human Genome Project was a $3 billion 13 year multi-center project to sequence human DNA. Humans have 23,000 genes, while rice has 45,000 genes. You mean, rice is more complex than humans? This puzzled the scientists until the Human Microbiome project (2007-2016) found 100 trillion microbes inhabiting the human gut with 500-1000 different strains of bacteria containing 3.3 million non-repeating genes. Hence, a human is mostly microbes, and our DNA blends with those of bacteria creating a complex organism called a human with 100 trillion voting "board members" in your gut. Killing the wrong bacteria in the gut creates the ultimate karma. We get to reap what we sow as poor health.

The microbiome is not limited to the gut. Studies have found that an individual's combination of bacteria also exists on the outside of the body, and even on surfaces the individual touches. We have microbes on our skin, lungs, sinuses, ears, vagina, and more. Altogether, you are more microbes than you.

Importance of a Healthy Microbiome

The microorganisms living in our bodies create a commensal (eating at the same dinner table) relationship that offers many health benefits to the host (you) and the microbes, hence symbiotic. We eat food, which is either digestible or indigestible (aka fiber, resistant starches, prebiotics). The fiber is digested by trillions of microbes in the gut yielding a daunting array of post-biotic compounds that can have powerful effects on our health.

Scientists involved in the Human Microbiome Project (2007-2016) were dazzled at the elegant and complex ways in which the 100 trillion organisms in our gut interact with our body. There is cross talk, or chemical messengers between the post biotics (by products of metabolism from the microbes) and the intestinal lumen. Gut Associated Lymphoid Tissue (GALT) and mucosal associated lymphoid tissue (MALT) showed scientists that up to 70% of the human immune system surrounds the gut, making gut health crucial for immune support. Then there is "quorum sensing" in which the balance of microbes swings the health of the gut in favor of illness or disease, not unlike an election in a democratic country. More bad guys than good guys spells trouble.

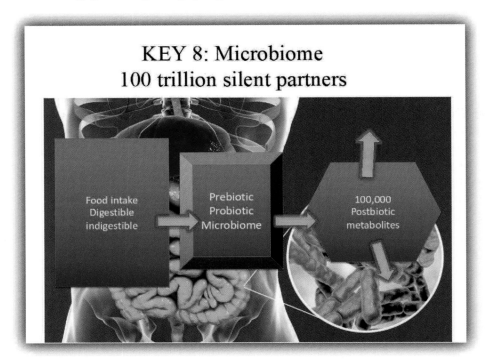

The microbiome acts like an additional organ with different functions in the body. The microbiome plays a part in almost 90 percent of diseases that affect us. The microbiome has a role in diseases and conditions like leaky gut syndrome, arthritis, heart disease, dementia, cancer, infertility and aging.

Magic or Science?

Studies with fecal microbiota transplants in animals have yielded dazzling results. Take the feces from calm animals and insert into the rectum of nervous animals, and the nervous animals become calm. Take the feces from obese animals and insert the feces into the rectum of lean animals and the leans animals become obese. And on it goes. This field of science is in its infancy and promises to reveal much about preventing and reversing disease in humans.

Microbiome Supports Digestion

While the human body produces enzymes to digest various types of food, different bacteria within the gut produce many more enzymes. This means that while the enzymes produced by the body have the capacity to digest a few types of food, microbiome enzymes can have a wider range of action. The result is that the bacteria make our bodies better equipped to access more nutrients from the food we eat. Which is why eating beans often upregulates or enhances the ability to digest the special starches in beans. Use it or lose it. The person who has beans only at the annual company picnic probably thinks that beans create an overabundance of flatulence, farting. But if you eat beans often, your microbiome obliges you by creating more enzymes to help digest beans properly.

Microbiome Lowers Inflammation

Some gut bacteria help to lower inflammation that may be caused by allergens and sensitivities to some foods and environmental components. This helps to reduce the effects of food and seasonal allergies and associated infections. When you have adequate friendly bacteria, your body is better equipped to resist inflammatory conditions and infections, including leaky gut syndrome, colds, coughs and sore throat. Many adverse food reactions are due to dysbiosis, or an unhappy gut.

Microbiome Can Help Boost immunity

A healthy gut with a higher ratio of friendly bacteria to harmful bacteria helps to support the immune system. This leads to better overall health and specifically protects against autoimmune conditions like arthritis, Hashimoto's disease and inflammatory bowel disease. In case of a higher ratio of harmful bacteria to friendly bacteria, autoimmune diseases are more likely to set in. It has been proven that excessive cleanliness in childhood is more likely to lead to autoimmune disease and allergies, aka the "hygiene hypothesis".[7]

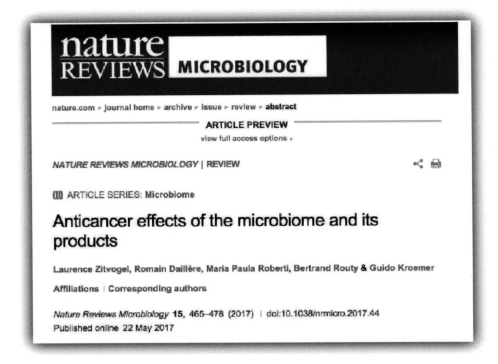

nature.com ► journal home ► archive ► issue ► review ► abstract

ARTICLE PREVIEW
view full access options ►

NATURE REVIEWS MICROBIOLOGY | REVIEW

(I0 ARTICLE SERIES: Microbiome

Anticancer effects of the microbiome and its products

Laurence Zitvogel, Romain Daillère, Maria Paula Roberti, Bertrand Routy & Guido Kroemer

Affiliations | Corresponding authors

Nature Reviews Microbiology 15, 465–478 (2017) | doi:10.1038/nrmicro.2017.44
Published online 22 May 2017

Promotes a Healthy Mind

Studies indicate that there are multiple nervous connections between the gut and the brain with signals being relayed back and forth. These signals are dependent on the composition of the gut microbiome and affect the mind in both short and long term. In case of poor gut microbiome balance, the signals from the gut may cause inflammation in parts of the brain and the nervous system. Such inflammation can lead to mental issues like poor memory, cognitive decline, dementia and Alzheimer's disease. When people talk about a "gut feeling" it is because we have a second brain in our gut.[8] Your gut influences the health of your mind. And your mind, e.g. stress, influences the health of your gut. The longest nerve in the body is the vagus nerve from the brain to the gut.

Mental health may depend on the creatures in your gut. What you eat or drink affects your gut microbiome. It also affects the activities of the neurotransmitters that are involved in the communication between the brain and the rest of the body systems. This affects how you feel. Research indicates that diet, lifestyle and environmental changes since the 20th century have led to increased depression and other emotional and mental health issues. This has been brought about by increased use of agricultural chemicals, depletion of nutrients due to over-farming and the resultant oxidative stress. These have affected levels of neurotransmitters like serotonin, dopamine and norepinephrine, which are responsible for mood changes.

Natasha Campbell-McBride, MD was a physician and neurologist who suddenly had a 2-year old autistic son. Nothing in the MD quiver of arrows can help autism. Dr. McBride researched other areas and found that most autistic children have a severe dysbiosis. Dr. McBride provided fermented foods plus whole animal foods with fat and was able to restore her autistic son to wellness, as documented in her book GUT AND PSYCHOLOGY SYNDROME.

Protects Against Cancers

Free radicals may have a role in the occurrence of cancer. Gut microorganisms are believed to influence human genes and cause or prevent inflammation and cancers. A healthy gut can quench free radicals and prevent cellular damage.

Microbes in the gut generate by-products such as butyrate, which is a powerful anti-cancer agent protecting colon cells. A healthy gut generates copious quantities of hydrogen gas, which is absorbed into the bloodstream and becomes a potent bioregulator, probably an essential nutrient. With dysbiosis comes a hydrogen deficiency, which provides antioxidant, anti-inflammatory, and regulatory action throughout the body. No wonder fiber deficiency creates such havoc with human health.

"The results revealed striking differences in fecal microbial population patterns between [colorectal cancer and healthy controls]."

Microb Ecol (2013) 66:462–470
DOI 10.1007/s00248-013-0245-9

HOST MICROBE INTERACTIONS

Dysbiosis Signature of Fecal Microbiota in Colorectal Cancer Patients

Na Wu · Xi Yang · Ruifen Zhang · Jun Li · Xue Xiao · Yongfei Hu · Yanfei Chen · Fengling Yang · Na Lu · Zhiyun Wang · Chunguang Luan · Yulan Liu · Baohong Wang · Charlie Xiang · Yuezhu Wang · Fangqing Zhao · George F. Gao · Shengyue Wang · Lanjuan Li · Haizeng Zhang · Baoli Zhu

Received: 24 December 2012 / Accepted: 3 May 2013 / Published online: 4 June 2013
© Springer Science+Business Media New York 2013

Abstract The human gut microbiota is a complex system that is essential to the health of the host. Increasing evidence suggests that the gut microbiota may play an important role in the pathogenesis of colorectal cancer (CRC). In this study, we used pyrosequencing of the 16S rRNA gene V3 region to characterize the fecal microbiota of 19 patients with CRC and differences in fecal microbial population patterns between these two groups. Partial least-squares discriminant analysis showed that 17 phylotypes closely related to *Bacteroides* were enriched in the gut microbiota of CRC patients, whereas nine operational taxonomic units, represented by the butyrate-producing genera *Faecalibacterium* and *Roseburia*, were sig-

What to Do?

Avoid:

- refined carbs, e.g. sugar, the "whites" rice, flour, potato
- excess animal protein and fats, especially trans fats (hydrogenated), which feed the unfriendly microbes in your gut.
- Hard liquor. Yeast ferment carbohydrates sources (grapes, hops, barley) into alcohol. At 15% alcohol (30 proof) the yeast begins to die. Hard liquor is 50-100% alcohol (=100-200 proof). If the creature that created the alcohol cannot live in it, then your body will suffer from exposure to extreme concentrations of alcohol. Hard liquor is close to antibiotics in purging the gut of friendly bacteria.

- Adverse food reactions. Many people react poorly to some foods. Then don't eat them. Wheat, dairy, nuts, eggs, shellfish, corn, and tomatoes are among the more common foods that cause problems in the gut. You can use the rotation method of determining food reactions or have your doctor do a food allergy test.
- Any unnecessary medications, especially antibiotics.
- Stress. There is a direct phone line from your brain to your gut and back. Worry, fear, depression etc. create havoc in the gut.

Include:

- Prebiotic-rich wholesome plant food which feeds the friendly microbes in your gut.
- Choose organic foods whenever possible to minimize exposure to glyphosate (Roundup).
- Consume fermented foods often, including yogurt, kimchi, sauerkraut, miso, and much more.
- Make sure that you have at least a daily bowel movement.
- Symptoms like diarrhea, gas, constipation, acid indigestion are indicators that something is wrong with your gut.
- Since making stomach acid at a pH of 2 is a billion fold change in pH from artery pH of 7.41, many people find that digestion improves by taking a tablespoon of vinegar or lemon juice or even fermented foods like sauerkraut with your meals.
- Get some professional help to fix gut problems. Betaine hydrochloride or digestive enzymes can be inexpensive ways to bolster your digestion.
- Since GERD (gastro esophageal reflux disorder) is so common and increases the risk for esophageal cancer 1300%, many people find relief by sleeping on a pillow wedge. I do.

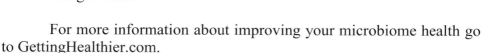

For more information about improving your microbiome health go to GettingHealthier.com.

PATIENT PROFILE

B.F. met with Dr. Quillin in May 2016. She was initially diagnosed with B-cell lymphoma. She was experienced problems with walking and visual disturbances. Initially B.F. was under the care of her oncologist and was doing chemotherapy per his recommendation. After her 6th chemotherapy session, and realizing the survival rate was limited, she began exploring other options. B.F. also underwent 2 Gamanite surgeries. Her oncologist told her the survival rate of those who have Gamanite surgery was 48%. At that time she first met with her local naturopath who gave her hope. Then, in 2016 she watched The Truth About Cancer and saw Dr. Quillin's presentation, and shortly after scheduled a consultation. Following her consultation with Dr. Quillin B.F. bought the book Beating Cancer with Nutrition, which she still uses as a reference book. She has made many changes to her lifestyle including; improved diet - though she has always had a reasonably healthy diet, more sunshine (Vitamin D), exercising 5X week, enjoys Tai Chi, has a green smoothie 3X week, has removed stress from her life, says a gratitude prayer every morning, and has read many books on healing cancer naturally. B.F.'s is very grateful for the advice from Dr. Quillin and credits him with the start in her holistic healing journey. Today B.F. is 69 feels great, has a grandchild on the way, and is looking forward to a long and healthy life.

ENDNOTES

[1] https://pdfs.semanticscholar.org/8b2c/6b5dcffe3a2f3e6c8dd494d560521d62feae.pdf
[2] https://www.ncbi.nlm.nih.gov/pubmed/28583217
[3] https://www.ncbi.nlm.nih.gov/pmc/articles/PMC3709439/
[4] https://www.sciencedirect.com/science/article/abs/pii/S1542356511008913
[5] https://www.cdc.gov/media/releases/2016/p0503-unnecessary-prescriptions.html
[6] https://www.amazon.com/Missing-Diagnosis-II-Dr-Truss/dp/0615273963
[7] https://www.ncbi.nlm.nih.gov/pmc/articles/PMC2841828/
[8] https://www.amazon.com/Second-Brain-Groundbreaking-Understanding-Disorders/dp/0060930721/ref=asc_df_0060930721/?tag=hyprod-20&linkCode=df0&hvadid=312031138203&hvpos=1o1&hvnetw=g&hvrand=15331521785663750767&hvpone=&hvptwo=&hvqmt=&hvdev=c&hvdvcmdl=&hvlocint=&hvlocphy=9031285&hvtargid=pla-448913064390&psc=1

KEY 9
NUTRITION

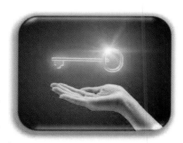

Chapter 9.0
You Are What You Eat

"Let food be your medicine and let medicine be your food."
Hippocrates, father of modern medicine 2400 years ago

FROM NATURE'S PHARMACY: Beetroot

If the soundbite "go for the color" has any merit, then beetroot should be near the top of the list for food choices. Most bioflavonoids and carotenoids are colorful pigments that participate in the process of photosynthesis. Beetroot "buries the needle" on color. Beetroot is a good source of fiber, vitamin C, iron, manganese, potassium and more. While some critics point out the simple carb content of beetroot, the glycemic load (taking into consideration the quality and quantity of carbohydrates) is a mere 5, very good. Mother Nature puts a root, like beets, in the ground with some sugar in it, and is surrounded by billions of fungi in the soil. The only way to protect that crop is with abundant anti-fungal compounds, which is a major benefit of whole cooked beetroot.

But the real magic with beetroot is in the inorganic nitrates. Nitrates in beetroot are wonderful precursors for nitric oxide in the body. In 1998 three scientists were awarded the Nobel Prize in Medicine for their discovery of nitric oxide as a signaling molecule in the cardiovascular system. Viagra for erectile dysfunction is 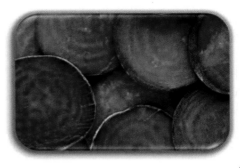 based on this principle of nitric oxide. Improving blood flow through enhanced nitric oxide has abundant health merits. As published in the American Journal of Clinical Nutrition, some very good scientists have proposed that nitrates in foods like beetroot be considered a nutrient for the incredible health benefits of enhanced circulation.[1]

Easiest recipe for beetroot: buy organic beets, clean, dice, place in pressure cooker, cover with a solution of 50:50 water and organic apple cider vinegar, pressure cook for 10 minutes. Eat often.

Nutrition is a crucial requirement for human health. It makes so much sense. And there is an abundance of evidence supporting the scientific link between optimal nutrition and optimal health. Every gardener and farmer knows that feeding the soil properly will make a huge difference in the vitality of the plants from the soil. Feeding animals in modern agriculture is a highly refined science, since there is no profit in sick animals as there is in sick humans. Nutrition scientists have created carefully crafted formulas for optimal health in chickens, pigs, cows, and other domestic animals. The scientists create pellets that have all the necessary macro and micronutrients so that the animal cannot spit out their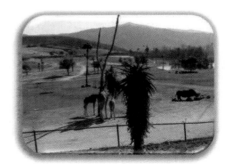

peas.   At the 1800-acre Wild Animal Park in San Diego where 2 million visitors per year view the 2600 animals on display, several scientists are employed to mimic the diet of the animals in the wild. If you deviate from the native indigenous diet of the animal, it will get sick.

Weston Price, DDS, was a dentist who began practicing around 1900. By 1930, Dr. Price noticed the dramatic deterioration in the oral health of his patients, with dental caries, crowded dentition (requiring wisdom teeth extraction), and periodontal disease. While most dentists would have been satisfied with that observation, Dr. Price asked the question "Does diet have anything to do with this deterioration in dental health?" Price and his wife, a nurse, travelled the world during the great depression, visiting 12 cultures on 5 continents and taking 15,000 photographs along with meticulous notes. Dr. Price observed that people within the same culture and same village eating different diets, one adhering to the native unprocessed diet and the other person embracing processed foods of white flour, sugar, and oils would develop dramatic differences in their jaw appearance as well as dental, physical, and mental

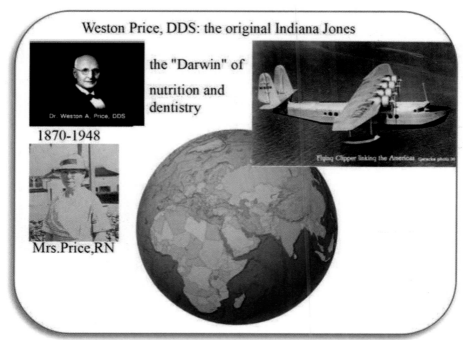

Weston Price, DDS: the original Indiana Jones

the "Darwin" of nutrition and dentistry

Dr. Weston A. Price, DDS

1870-1948

Mrs.Price,RN

Flying Clipper linking the Americas

health. Price's 1939 book, NUTRITION AND PHYSICAL DEGENERATION, was one of the earliest works documenting the health costs of deviating from our native indigenous diet. Price found that processed foods created enormous problems in dental, physical and mental health.

Today Americans spend $111 billion per year on dental work, with about $4 billion of that spent on dental implants. While a huge issue in political campaigns revolves around "who is going to pay for my health care bills?", no one has asked for free dental work along with national medicare.

While there are thousands of legitimate scientific studies in peer reviewed journals supporting the efficacy and safety of nutrition for healing, only the few negative studies are reported in the mainstream media. That's because Big Pharma spends $6 billion advertising drugs to the public and another $20 billion schmoozing docs. Your TV station will not promote nutrition supplements as a solution for health problems when their primary source of income is drug company TV ads.

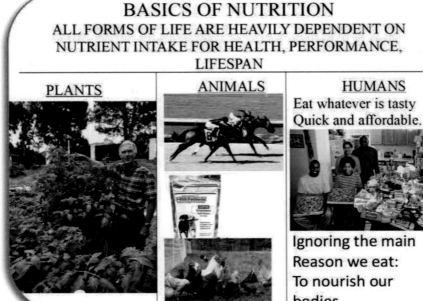

BASICS OF NUTRITION
ALL FORMS OF LIFE ARE HEAVILY DEPENDENT ON NUTRIENT INTAKE FOR HEALTH, PERFORMANCE, LIFESPAN

PLANTS	ANIMALS	HUMANS
		Eat whatever is tasty Quick and affordable.

Ignoring the main Reason we eat: To nourish our bodies

Many of the negative studies on nutrition supplements ignore the basics of biochemistry. Nutrients are molecules with a three-dimensional structure, like a house key. Nutrients cannot be tweaked into a mild variation and have the results the same. It's not nice to fool with Mother Nature. The difference between a man and woman, other than the genetic XX or XY chromosome, is hormones. The difference between the male hormone, testosterone, and female hormone, estradiol, is a 3 tiny OH groups on an otherwise identical molecule. Tiny differences in chemical structure make a huge difference in activity in the body.

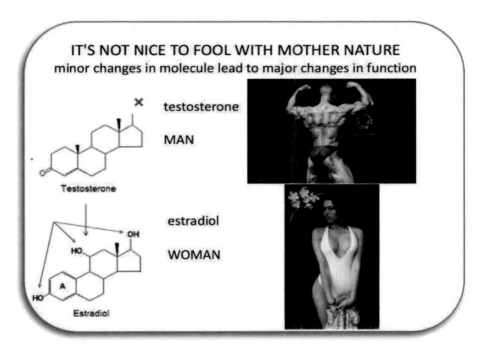

One of the problems in proving the efficacy of nutritional medicine is the tenacity of humans. Humans are hard to kill. You might need to smoke for 40 years before lung cancer crops up. You might eat poorly for decades before a serious illness is diagnosed. Humans are built to survive. But we can only thrive, live longer, delay, reverse or prevent disease by employing optimal nutrition.

Hippocrates is considered the founder of modern medicine 2400 years ago. Hippocrates was a nutritionist and herbalist. The Hippocratic oath taken by modern medical doctors includes the following passage:
"I will use treatment to help the sick according to my ability and judgment, but never with a view to injury and wrong-doing."

Of the $38 billion annual budget at the National Institutes of Health, allegedly $1.5 billion is spent on nutrition research. The vast majority of government funding for science goes to research that will eventually produce a patentable FDA approved drug. We study ways to palliate the symptoms of illness, but rarely ways to maintain health or prevent disease, especially through the obvious modality of nutrition.

The link between nutrition and health is blatantly seen in pregnancy. Mother and baby suffer if nutritional status is poor. Which is why <u>Vitamin Angels</u> delivers prenatal nutrition supplements to 70 million mothers and children in 70 countries around the world. Because you never get a second chance to make a baby. Nutrition deficiencies can make the difference in having a child that is healthy and bright, or has some birth defect or is mentally retarded.

The data on "evidence based" nutrition science is staggering. Alan Gaby, MD is a physician and biochemical nutritionist whose 40 years of clinical practice combined with 15,000 peer reviewed references makes up his tome **<u>NUTRITIONAL MEDICINE</u>**. Melvyn Werbach, MD has compiled a separate review of the world's literature on using nutrition supplements and foods to prevent and reverse many common ailments in **<u>NUTRITIONAL INFLUENCES ON ILLNESS</u>**. Sheldon Hendler, MD, PhD has authored the **<u>PHYSICIANS DESK REFERENCE OF NUTRITIONAL SUPPLEMENTS</u>**. Michael Murray, ND and Joseph Pizzorno, ND have authored **<u>ENCYCLOPEDIA OF NATURAL MEDICINE</u>**, another fine reference book for this field. Life Extension has compiled a 3800 page massive textbook **<u>DISEASE PREVENTION AND TREATMENT</u>** which uses largely nutrition protocols to reverse 131 common ailments. We could go on.

The point is: there is overwhelming evidence showing that nutrition protocols are logical, humane, scientific and need to be included as front-line therapy. In truth, few medical schools teach any nutrition, and most of the 900,000 medical doctors in American are highly ignorant or sarcastic of nutrition therapies. Many a good doctor has lost his/her medical license or been chased out of a state by a fiercely protective medical board seeking "standard of care", read: drugs and surgery.

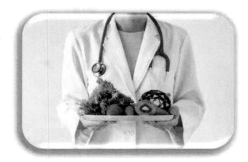

Without health nothing else matters. Our health bill is huge and unsustainable. With current trends in diabetes, obesity, cancer, kidney disease, heart disease, mental illness, Alzheimer's disease etc., we will soon be at a breaking point, even with an unlimited checking account. We must begin to use rational therapies, which starts with nutrition as the fulcrum for lifestyle changes. Nutrition as front line therapy is evidence-based, efficient, economical, humane, and irreplaceable. Nutrition is true 21st century medicine.

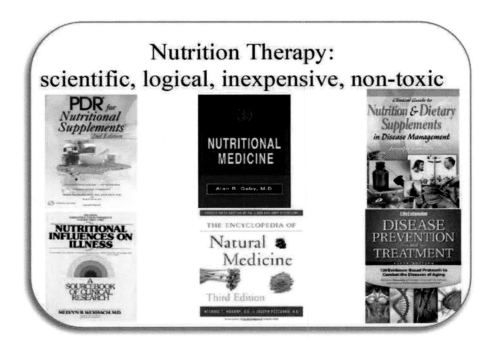

For more information on nutrition go to GettingHealthier.com.

PATIENT PROFILE: BEAT PANCREATIC CANCER.

RM was diagnosed with advanced adenocarcinoma of the pancreas in August 1996 at the age of 53. His lifestyle was unhealthy. He was obese and on cholesterol lowering drugs. His doctors admitted that this cancer was a "poor prognostic" cancer, meaning very few people beat the condition. RM underwent surgery (Whipple), chemo, and radiation. He felt sorry for himself briefly, then realized that he was going to do everything in his power to beat this cancer, including a fighting spirit. RM followed the advice in BEATING CANCER WITH NUTRITION, including food, supplements, and eating your way through the nausea of intra-arterial infusion chemo. He kept the subclavian port (medical device that allows doctors to inject chemo into the vein near the neck) in place for another 7 years to remind himself of his newfound healthier lifestyle. As of February 2010, and at 66 years of age, RM was in complete remission, travels the world, feels great, and doesn't worry anymore. Cancer has brought RM a newfound sense of "life is short and precious, savor it, and do not worry your way through it." His doctors were very pleased and surprised at RM's admirable outcome.

ENDNOTES

[1] https://academic.oup.com/ajcn/article/90/1/1/4596750

KEY 9
NUTRITION

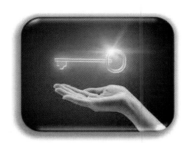

Chapter 9.1
Malnutrition USA

"Americans are digging their graves with spoons and forks."

<u>**FROM NATURE'S PHARMACY: *Resveratrol***</u>

In spite of a high fat diet, the French have had a relatively low incidence of heart disease. Labeled the "French paradox", there is compelling evidence that resveratrol, found in red wine and other foods, may lower the risk for heart disease, cancer, diabetes, Alzheimer's and even slow the aging process. Resveratrol is found in the skin of red grapes and is produced by a few plants as a defense against attacking bacteria or fungi. All trans resveratrol (as compared to all cis-resveratrol) is the preferred and more active form of this substance. Some research finds that resveratrol may actually affect the genes (Sirtuin 1) that slow the aging process, just like calorie restriction. Resveratrol has demonstrated some activity at regulating blood glucose, preventing or slowing cancer growth, improving exercise capacity, and preventing the formation of plaques in the brain that cause Alzheimer's disease. Resveratrol is a polyphenol, which is an important class of phytochemicals. Other foods that are rich in polyphenols that have demonstrated health benefits include green tea, dark chocolate, 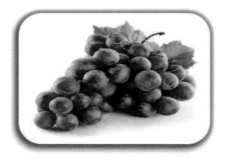 pomegranates, apples and berries. Enjoy organic red grapes often. Use 100% frozen grape juice concentrate as a liquid base for pureed whole fruit and veggie drinks. Or use red wine in moderation at dinnertime.

It is hard to believe that there can be malnutrition in this agriculturally abundant nation of ours--but there is. "Poor food choices" summarizes our dilemma at the dinner table. America is blessed to have enough food, but we are eating the wrong food and too much of it and too often. Food manufacturers know your palate better than you. The fast food industry has grown from annual sales of $6 billion in 1970 to $200 billion in 2015. Add in the junk food and beverages that clogs the aisles at the grocery and liquor stores and you have a trillion dollar a year industry that makes many consumers like a moth to a flame…the food (flame) looks and tastes good, but will kill you.

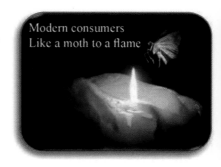

Modern consumers
Like a moth to a flame

From Lean Farmers to Obese Commuters

At the time of the Revolutionary War, 96% of Americans farmed while only 4% worked at other trades. Tractors and harvesting combines became part of an agricultural revolution that allowed the 2% of Americans who now farm to feed the rest of us. We grow enough food in this country (quantity) to feed ourselves, to make 2/3 of us overweight, to throw away enough food to feed 50 million people daily, to ship food overseas as a major export, and to store enough food in government surplus bins to feed Americans for a year if all farmers quit today. With so much food available, how can Americans be malnourished?

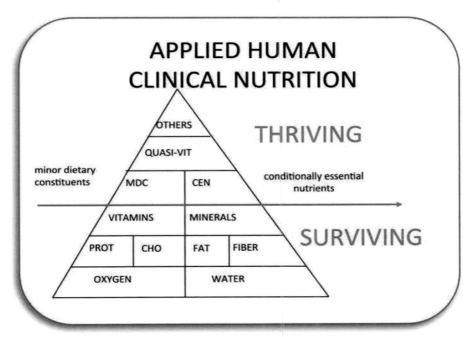

Among the many tragedies in the western diet is the ignorance of basic math in fertilizing the soil. There are 118 elements in the periodic table, the building blocks of the planet earth. Of those 118, about 83 are considered possibly important in human and plant health. Of those 83 only 15 are considered essential in the human diet. Of those 15 only 3 are added to the soil (nitrogen, potassium, phosphorus...NPK) in agribusiness. As a result of this myopic approach to soil fertilizing, the USDA has documented a 60% decline in the mineral content of many American produce items.

Among the many tragedies in the western diet is the ignorance of basic math in fertilizing the soil. There are 118 elements in the periodic table, the building blocks of the planet earth. Of those 118, about 83 are considered possibly important in human and plant health. Of those 83 only 15 are considered essential in the human diet. Of those 15 only 3 are added to the soil (nitrogen, potassium, phosphorus...NPK) in agribusiness. As a result of this myopic approach to soil fertilizing, the USDA has documented a 60% decline in the mineral content of many American produce items.

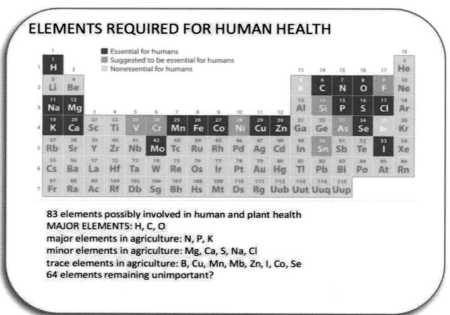

ELEMENTS REQUIRED FOR HUMAN HEALTH

83 elements possibly involved in human and plant health
MAJOR ELEMENTS: H, C, O
major elements in agriculture: N, P, K
minor elements in agriculture: Mg, Ca, S, Na, Cl
trace elements in agriculture: B, Cu, Mn, Mb, Zn, I, Co, Se
64 elements remaining unimportant?

Americans choose their food based upon taste, cost, convenience, and psychological gratification--thus ignoring the main reason that we eat, which is to provide our body cells with the raw materials to grow, repair, and fuel our bodies. The most commonly eaten foods in America are white bread, coffee, and hot dogs. The most commonly consumed fruits and vegetables, according to the USDA, is catsup, French fries, and onion rings. Based upon our food abundance, Americans could be the best nourished nation on record. But we are far from it.

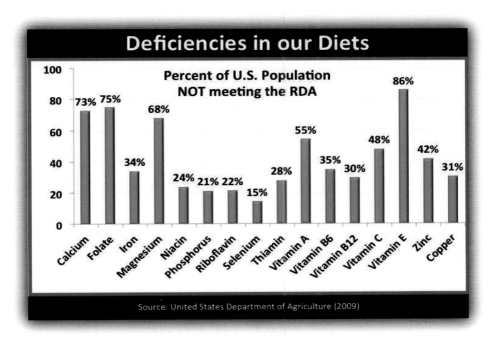

Causes of Nutrient Deficiencies

There are many reasons for developing malnutrition:

⇒ We don't eat well due to poor food choices, loss of appetite, discomfort in the gastrointestinal region, or consuming nutritionally bankrupt "junk food"; many people just don't get enough nutrients into their stomachs.

⇒ We don't absorb nutrients due to loss of digestive functions (including low hydrochloric acid or enzyme output), allergy, "leaky gut", or intestinal infections, like yeast overgrowth.

⇒ We don't keep enough nutrients due to increased excretion or loss of nutrients because of diarrhea, vomiting, or drug interactions.

⇒ We don't get enough nutrients due to increased requirements caused by fever, disease, alcohol, or drug interactions.

Anyone who is confused about why we spend so much on medical care with such poor results in cancer treatment might glean some wisdom by reading what sells best in American grocery stores.

Overwhelming evidence from both government and independent scientific surveys shows that many Americans are low in their intake of a wide variety of nutrients:

- VITAMINS: A, D, E, C, B-6, riboflavin, folacin, pantothenic acid.
- MINERALS: calcium, potassium, magnesium, zinc, iron, chromium, selenium; and possibly molybdenum and vanadium.
- MACRONUTRIENTS: fiber, complex carbohydrates, plant protein, special fatty acids (EPA, GLA, ALA), clean water.

Meanwhile, we also eat alarmingly high amounts of: fat, salt, sugar, cholesterol, alcohol, caffeine, food additives, and toxins.

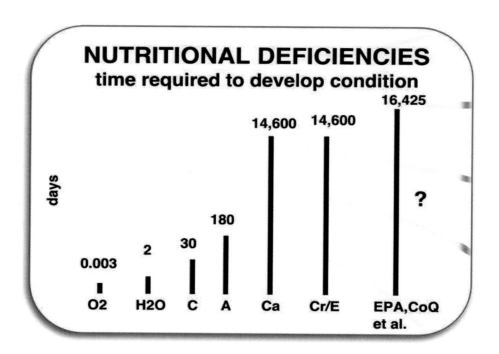

This combination of too much of the wrong things along with not enough of the right things has created epidemic proportions of degenerative diseases in this country. The Surgeon General, Department of Health and Human Services, Center for Disease Control, National Academy of Sciences, American Medical Association, American Dietetic Association, and others agree that diet is a major contributor to our most common health problems. Nutritional deficiencies oftentimes do not manifest quickly. Some take years before a long term subclinical deficiency of a nutrient explodes as a major disease, such as osteoporosis, cancer, heart disease, diabetes, and more.

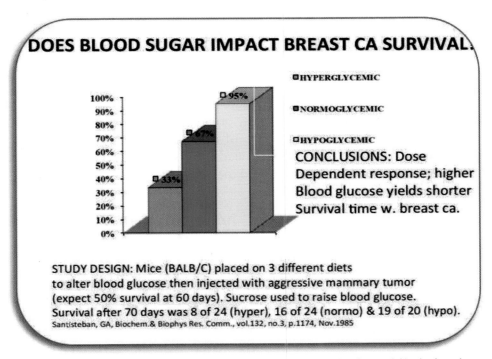

DOES BLOOD SUGAR IMPACT BREAST CA SURVIVAL?

☐ HYPERGLYCEMIC

☐ NORMOGLYCEMIC

☐ HYPOGLYCEMIC

CONCLUSIONS: Dose Dependent response; higher Blood glucose yields shorter Survival time w. breast ca.

STUDY DESIGN: Mice (BALB/C) placed on 3 different diets to alter blood glucose then injected with aggressive mammary tumor (expect 50% survival at 60 days). Sucrose used to raise blood glucose. Survival after 70 days was 8 of 24 (hyper), 16 of 24 (normo) & 19 of 20 (hypo). Santisteban, GA, Biochem.& Biophys Res. Comm., vol.132, no.3, p.1174, Nov.1985

The typical diet of the cancer patient is high in fat, while being low in fiber and vegetables--"meat, potatoes, and gravy" is what many of my patients lived on. Data collected by the United States Department of Agriculture from over 11,000 Americans showed that on any given day:

- 41% did not eat any fruit
- 82% did not eat cruciferous vegetables
- 72% did not eat vitamin C-rich fruits or vegetables
- 80% did not eat vitamin A-rich fruits or vegetables
- 84% did not eat high fiber grain food, like bread or cereal

Sugar

The average American consumes 150 lb/yr of refined sugars. 30 million Americans are diabetic with another 60 million as prediabetic, or ticking time bombs. Too much sugar in the diet, the gut, and the blood is killing Americans. The nearby study found a dose dependent response: the higher the blood glucose of these animals with implanted tumors, the shorter the lifespan. Refined sugar kills.

Native Human Diet

Our ancestor's (Paleolithic) diet was dramatically different than our current Standard American Diet, or SAD. If we ever hope to get a handle on our epidemic proportions of disease then we need to start by addressing our body's nutrient needs through a pristine (organic, biodynamic), whole food, plant based diet.

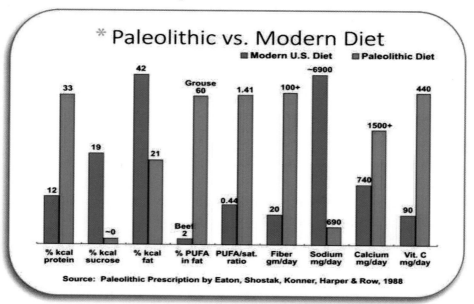

*Paleolithic vs. Modern Diet

Source: Paleolithic Prescription by Eaton, Shostak, Konner, Harper & Row, 1988

For more information on malnutrition in the USA go to GettingHealthier.com.

PATIENT PROFILE:

T.S. arrived on our hospital doorstep as a "medical emergency" in an ambulance. At age 53, he had been treated at a previous hospital for stage 4 lymphoma and failed therapy. Our team quickly realized that T.S. was dying from both cancer and malnutrition. Since he could not eat, we provided TPN (total parenteral nutrition) through his subclavian vein for a month, then got him on a good diet, then he was capable of tolerating our fractionated chemotherapy. Within 6 months, he was in complete remission. I saw him 7 years later and he was looking fabulous.

KEY 9
NUTRITION

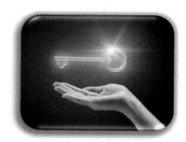

Chapter 9.2
Nutrition as Frontline Therapy

"Germs do not cause disease in the real sense. Something happens in the body to allow the germs to become invasive."
Antoine Bechamp, MD, PhD circa 1900

FROM NATURE'S PHARMACY: Pigmented Potatoes

Potatoes were indigenous to the high Andes mountains in South America. Brought back to Europe in 1536 by the Spanish explorers, scientists ruled the potato unfit for human consumption. So the Irish grew potatoes abundantly, which doubled the population, which led to a catastrophe when the potato crop was devastated by a blight in 1845, leading to the death from starvation and migration of millions of Irish throughout the world. My ancestors were among them.

There is a huge difference between the generic white potato and pigmented potatoes. White potatoes are GMO, high in glycemic index and very low in phytochemicals. Pigmented potatoes (orange, purple) are low in glycemic index, very high in phytochemicals and not GMO. In 2006 the world's oldest human, Benito Martinez, died in Cuba at the age of 126. His diet consisted primarily of sweet potatoes grown in his backyard. Several Asian cultures are known for their longevity and thrive on purple potatoes.

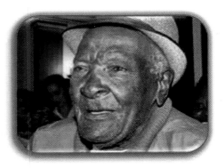

One baked sweet potato provides a decent meal with protein, vitamin C, abundant A, fiber, manganese, B-6, potassium, pantothenic acid, copper, niacin. The real magic in the pigmented potatoes is the panoply of bioflavonoids and carotenoids that serve

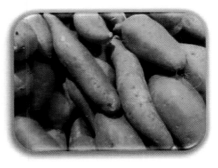

as <u>**antioxidants, anti-aging, anti-cancer**</u> compounds in your body.[1] Bake or pressure cook, then add a little butter, olive oil, nut meal and you have a delicious and nutritious meal.

Most of human nutrition throughout time and the entire planet has involved just getting enough to eat. Yet bright minds often pondered the subject of nutrition. What is in foods? Why do we need to eat to live? What do these food components do in our bodies? How do we eat a steak or carrot and turn that food into part of our body? All good questions.

In 1913 Casimir Funk coined the phrase "vital amine" to represent the idea that something in food, in this case thiamin from rice bran, was able to cure a condition in chickens. By 1926, thiamin, or vitamin B1 had been synthesized and the race for answers in the science of nutrition was on. In general, scientists sought to couple a nutrient with a deficiency syndrome, such as vitamin C and scurvy. It was assumed that if you had no frank blatant clinical deficiency of a nutrient, then you must be well nourished.

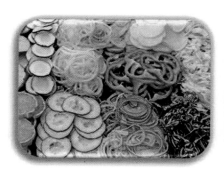

Until the New York Academy of Sciences published their textbook on "Beyond Deficiencies". [2] Just because a person cannot be diagnosed with a frank clinical nutritional deficiency, does not mean that person is well nourished. Nutrients at higher than survival doses take on meta-nutrient capabilities and work throughout the body to provide optimal health as opposed to just keeping the person alive.

META NUTRIENT FUNCTIONS: BEYOND DEFICIENCY

VITAMIN D:
    400 iu prev. rickets
    2000-10,000 iu regulate 20% genome, prev.diseases
VITAMIN K:
    120 mcg/d prevent hemorrhaging
    500+ mcg/d improves bone health, cancer prev.

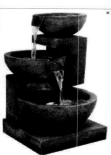

VITAMIN C: 60 mg/d prev.scurvy
90 mg/d lowers risk endom ca.
1000 mg/d enhances wound heal
FOLATE: 400 mcg/d avoid meg. anemia
10,000 mcg reverse dysplasia
30,000 mcg vasodilator, lo blood p.
NIACIN: 20 mg prev.pellagra
100 mg vasodilator
2000 mg lowers cholesterol

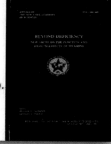

Frontline Therapy?

Modern physicians use drugs and surgery as frontline therapies in 99% of their patients. Foods are considered less scientific and less targeted. Many a physician has lost his/her medical license for using nutrition as front line therapy...the first therapy to be considered when a patient is ill.

There are many reasons why nutrition should be considered front line therapy:

1) *Basic nutrition*. You are what you eat. Your body is composed of nutrients consumed over your lifetime. Your body is built from, repaired by, regulated by, and fueled by the nutrients in your diet. There are basic macronutrients (protein, carbohydrate, fat, fiber, water) and micronutrients (vitamins, minerals) that are taught in all approved nutrition courses around the world. But there is more to nutrition than this basic need.

2) *Beyond deficiencies*. While 10 mg/day of vitamin C will prevent scurvy in most adults, 90 mg/day will lower the risk for various cancers by 50%, and 1000 mg/day will help to reduce bleeding and bruising in older adults. Beyond deficiencies demonstrates that many nutrients take on meta-nutrient functions when provided at beyond survival dosages. Bruce Ames, PhD at the University of California Berkeley has shown that long term <u>low intake of various nutrients creates fragile DNA</u>, which eventually leads to cancer and/or premature aging. There is a huge difference between surviving and thriving financially, emotionally, physically, and nutritionally.

3) *Quasi nutrients*. There are conditionally essential nutrients found throughout our food supply that are not considered essential for survival but have been shown to be incredibly useful at preventing or reversing common ailments. Coenzyme Q, lipoic acid, EPA and DHA from fish oil, sulforaphane and DIM from broccoli, bioflavonoids and carotenoids in abundance from fresh fruits and vegetables, ellagic acid in dark berries, lycopenes in tomatoes. And on it goes. In order to survive long enough to have two children and keep your DNA in the gene pool, you can eat almost

anything that keeps you alive. If you want to thrive beyond those 20 years, then you need to be more cautious about your nutrient intake.

4) ***Information***. RNA and DNA in food can be absorbed into the bloodstream and <u>turn on or off various DNA mechanisms</u>. Food is information telling your body how to function. Cartilage contains "bioregulators" that work to dampen down abnormal growth. John Prudden, MD, PhD founded the field of bovine cartilage for cancer. The evidence cannot be ignored that <u>cartilage seems to help the body function better</u>.

5) ***Energy***. Now it really gets into future thinking. All of the universe is nothing more than pulsing energy. Quantum mechanics has rewritten the books on physics. Energy can be released from a small cube of uranium to power a nuclear submarine or demolish a city. All of the sciences can be reduced to equations on energy. The human body is an incredibly complex, tenacious, and fragile energy generator. Food has energy and a quantum fingerprint of its life force. That said, if a food will not rot or sprout, then throw it out. Dead food cannot provide you with life.

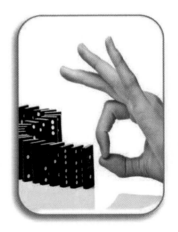

Malnutrition is often the beginning domino to fall, ending in some poor prognostic condition, like late stage cancer. The only solution for malnutrition is optimal nutrition. No drug can take the place of essential nutrients for your body.

For more information about frontline therapy for cancer patients go to <u>GettingHealthier.com</u>.

PATIENT PROFILE

S.R. was diagnosed at age 48 with stage 4 non-Hodgkins B-cell lymphoma. Tumor was the size of a potato and choking off blood to the intestines. Underwent chemo regimen. S.R. used nutrition supplements in spite of oncologist's hostility to the subject. S.R. was able to work throughout chemo, travelling to trade shows, though he did lose his hair. Four years later S.R. was in complete remission and has learned the value of good nutrition, living more joyfully, and faith in God.

ENDNOTES

[1] https://www.hindawi.com/journals/ijfs/2016/3631647/abs/
[2] https://www.amazon.com/Beyond-Deficiency-Function-Vitamins-Sciences/dp/0897667506

KEY 9
NUTRITION

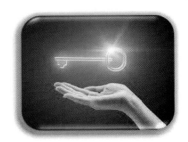

Chapter 9.3
Real Food and Healing
What is Real Food and Why Does it Matter?

"Each patient carries his own doctor inside him."
Albert Schweitzer, MD, Nobel laureate, 1940

FROM NATURE'S PHARMACY: Seaweed

There are thousands of species of edible plants on earth, of which a couple dozen of those plant foods make it to your local grocery store. Same thing happens in the ocean. There are hundreds of different sea vegetables, or seaweed, technically microalgae. There are 3 types of seaweed, based on how deep the water in which the plant grows. Green seaweed grows in shallow water and has the characteristic green chlorophyll for photosynthesis. Brown seaweed grows in deeper water and still conducts photosynthesis, but with different colored pigments. Red seaweed grows in even deeper water and has specially adapted to perform photosynthesis with the meager light it receives.

Seaweed is rich in protein, some vitamins, fiber, and a fabulous source of iodine as well as other trace minerals found in the ocean and probably useful to your body. At least <u>2 billion people suffer</u> from an iodine deficiency.[1] While seaweed tastes salty, it is actually low in sodium, but very high in potassium, which gives it the salty taste. Nori, wakame, and dulse are some common seaweed varieties found in American stores. Seaweed is rich in bioflavonoids, carotenoids, and an ingredient of particular interest fucoxanthin, or fucoidan. Seaweed provides a plethora of nutrients that are <u>antioxidants, anti-inflammatory, anti-cancer, anti-obesity</u>, and more.[2]

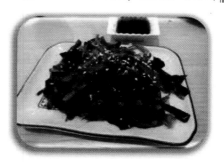

Japan has one of the lowest incidences of cancer in the world. The Japanese people consider seaweed to be a daily staple in their diet. In Oriental restaurants you can buy a bowl of green seaweed that is delicious. Or buy the dried seaweed, which tastes a little bit like green potato chips. Enjoy!

Your body is the most amazing organism on earth. 37 trillion cells each performing 100,000 chemical reactions per second. Lungs with the surface area of a tennis court that bring in 11,000 liters of air per day that circulates oxygen through the 60,000 miles of blood vessels to feed each cell and carry away the waste products of living. Your brain has 100 billion cells with each of them having 1000 connections to other brain cells, making 100 trillion junctions in the brain for memory. Your gut includes a dazzling array of digestive enzymes, bile salts, and 100 trillion microorganisms to help in the process. All of this occurs on auto-pilot. If you are not at least a little bit impressed, then you are not paying attention.

And all of this grand symphony of life occurs because of what you eat. Your body is built from, repaired by, regulated by, and fueled by your diet. For better or worse, what you eat will greatly influence your quality and quantity of life. If you don't have your health, then nothing else really matters. If you can regain and retain good health through a diet of real food, then let's get started.

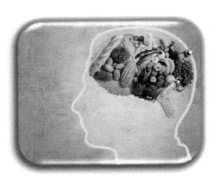

All of life is built around nutrition. Most religions have prescriptions (eat it) and proscriptions (don't eat it) about food. The first mono-theistic religion, Judaism, assigned an important task to the Rabbis in monitoring the purity of the food supply and the humane raising and slaughtering of animals. Fasting was the beginning of the ministry for all

"Better living through chemistry." DuPont Chemical 1935-82

Nutrition experiments:
1. milling of grain, white flour, 1000 AD Europe
2. beri-beri, 1897
3. saturated fat in butter to hydrogenated fats in margarine, trans vs cis fats
4. high fructose corn syrup
5. genetically modified organisms: GMO

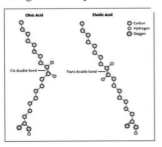

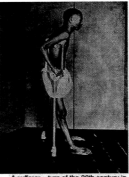

A sufferer – turn of the 20th century in

great spiritual leaders throughout history. The recent triple crown winner, Destiny, was fed a very particular diet dictated by its trainer. Farmers know the importance of feeding your soil properly in order to get an abundant harvest. Every major zoo on earth employs a scientist schooled in the art of feeding captive animals exactly what they ate in the wild. When obesity first became a problem, a famous adage was "we dig our graves with our teeth". With all the logic and science behind nutrition, modern humans instead select whatever food is convenient, tasty, and cheap; thus ignoring the primary reason for eating...to feed this extraordinary organism of your body.

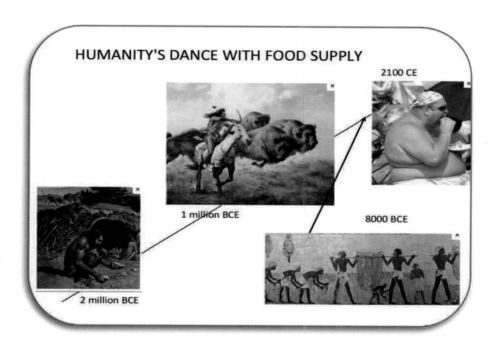

OOPS

What if you got the answers to the final exam before the test? Would you use them? Here are the answers. Mother Nature knows best. Review the chapter on the "Adaptive Forces of Nature". For millennium, humans have been tampering with our food supply, nearly always with disastrous results. Were it not for junk food, we would have no nutrition science. Yes, millions died and suffered in the process, but let's get to the point.

Food processors found that grinding wheat separated the chaff (bran and germ) from the grain (white flour). By around 1100 AD, England was awash in grain grinders because white flour produced bread that was "tastier" and had a longer shelf life, because all the life in the whole wheat was separated in the grinding process. Although the two greatest civilizations on earth, Egypt and Rome, used whole wheat as their staples, wheat as we see it today is not the same. Stripping the bran and germ from wheat was one of the greatest robberies on earth, causing the premature death of tens of millions of people. The greater the accuracy of our laboratory equipment, the more scientists can "see" into the various quasi vitamins that make whole food such a treasure trove of health.

Wheat

Around 1820, Reverend Sylvester Graham found that feeding people whole wheat, created meaningful bowel movements and significant relief from health problems caused by chronic constipation. His idea eventually led to Graham crackers and a food industry. The Kellogg brothers found that whole grain corn could relieve many health conditions, just by producing a daily bowel movement. The Kellogg food company was born around 1922 on this principle. Still, after centuries of nutrition scientists assuring the public that fiber cannot be digested and therefore was better off eliminated from food, the plagues of civilization continued. "We are taking this waste product out of your food for your own good. You are welcome."

Rice

Around 1895, Christiaan Eikjman was a Dutch physician sent to Indonesia to resolve the disease known as "beriberi", literally "I cannot, I cannot." Locals in Indonesia eating the processed white rice, compliments of the Dutch milling machines, developed a condition of weakness and eventually heart failure. About 30,000 people died with many more developing polio like symptoms. Eikjman eventually discovered that eating the "garbage" of the milling process, meaning the rice bran, cured beriberi. At the time, no one could conceive of something in food curing or preventing any health condition. In 1929, Dr. Eikjman was awarded the shared Nobel Prize in Medicine. Were it not for processing of real food into junk food (white rice), then the science of nutrition would not have been born.

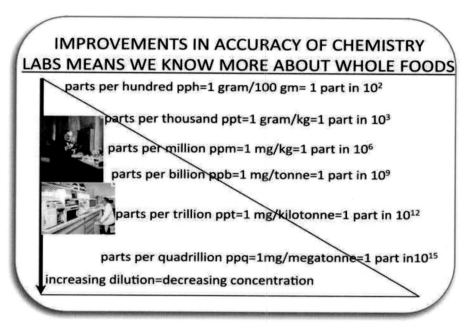

IMPROVEMENTS IN ACCURACY OF CHEMISTRY LABS MEANS WE KNOW MORE ABOUT WHOLE FOODS

parts per hundred pph=1 gram/100 gm= 1 part in 10^2

parts per thousand ppt=1 gram/kg=1 part in 10^3

parts per million ppm=1 mg/kg=1 part in 10^6

parts per billion ppb=1 mg/tonne=1 part in 10^9

parts per trillion ppt=1 mg/kilotonne=1 part in 10^{12}

parts per quadrillion ppq=1mg/megatonne=1 part in10^{15}

increasing dilution=decreasing concentration

Citrus

Albert Szent-Györgyi, MD, PhD earned the Nobel Prize in Medicine in 1937 for his work on vitamin C. Yet, his real passion was for the unidentified factor, eventually called flavonoids, in citrus fruits. Tang was a fruit flavored drink formulated by General Foods and sent to the moon in 1969. Tang consisted of sugar, vitamin C, and fruit flavorings…woefully lacking in the thousands of other nutrients in a real orange.

Not until the Human Microbiome Project was completed in 2017 could scientists confirm that because fiber was indigestible it was essential. Among the many benefits of feeding our microbiome with fiber is the production of butyrate, a powerful anti-cancer substance that feeds the intestinal mucosa. Mother Nature has not made any mistakes here. It was poetry in design.

Trans Fats

Margarine was invented in France at Napoleon's request for a cheap butter substitute for the soldiers. In those days, beef tallow was used to make margarine. During World War II, there was a shortage of farmers who went to war, and a shortage of butter for the troops. Nutrition scientists went to work, developing and marketing margarine which was made from soy, corn, or safflower oil that had been hydrogenated. The chemical formula was the same as a saturated fat, yet the 3 dimensional shape of the molecule changed from nature's "cis" (looks like a horseshoe) to "trans" (looks like a lightning bolt). Try bending your house key even slightly and see how well it works in your front door lock. Same thing happened with trans fats, which are directly related to risk for heart

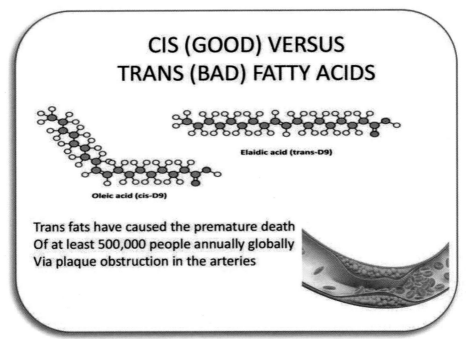

CIS (GOOD) VERSUS TRANS (BAD) FATTY ACIDS

Elaidic acid (trans-D9)

Oleic acid (cis-D9)

Trans fats have caused the premature death Of at least 500,000 people annually globally Via plaque obstruction in the arteries

disease, causing the premature deaths of <u>500,000 people globally</u> annually.[3]

Phytic Acid

In the 1960s nutrition scientists discovered phytic acid in whole grains, legumes, and seeds. This phytic acid seemed to be an "anti-nutrient", since it had strong binding capacity to minerals. Food scientists were eager to remove the fiber, along with the phytic acid, since clearly Mother Nature made a mistake here. Upon further research, the scientists found the phytic acid, now sold as a nutrition supplement IP6 (inositol hexaphosphate 6), actually has extraordinary healing capacities, with pharmacological benefits throughout the body, including <u>anti-cancer activity</u>. Their conclusions were:

"Given the numerous health benefits, phytates... inclusion as an essential nutrient, perhaps a vitamin."[4]

Mother's Milk

Mother's milk is another classic example of arrogance and ignorance attempting to improve on Mother Nature. In the 1950s, doctors discouraged new mother's from breastfeeding, citing the thin runny early milk as inadequate to nourish a newborn infant. In fact, that "runny stuff" is colostrum, a rich soup of immune factors designed to protect the newborn infant from the many assaults on this immature immune system. Fortunately, women prevailed, and up to 77% of new mother's now 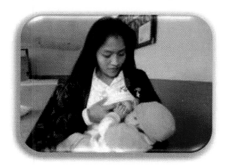 breastfeed their infants. To this day, there are many examples of the inferiority of infant formulas vs breast milk. To this day, the first ingredient in infant formula is high fructose corn syrup, a substance known to cause diabetes, heart disease, fatty liver disease, and more.

As mentioned in the section on Adaptive Forces of Nature, real whole milk from free range animals is a very different food from the pasteurized, homogenized milk from animals kept confined and fed GMO corn along with antibiotics and hormones to gain weight faster. Commercial milk increases the risk for prostate cancer. Small amounts of cheese, yogurt, and butter might slightly reduce the risk for cancer. Free range cheese from goats helps the people in Ikaria, Greece live to 90.

Meat

Same thing goes for meat. Our ancestors ate small amounts of free range animals. Humans get sick without exercise. So do animals. Obese humans are sick. So are obese animals. It is not wise to eat a sick animal that has been living a very unnatural lifestyle.

Follow the Money Trail

If real food is so healing, then why doesn't my doctor tell me about it and the mainstream media feature stories about? Good questions. See the chapter on "If This Stuff Works…" Sickness management in America is a $3.5 trillion/year industry, including $440 billion in drugs. It is difficult to advertise broccoli or peaches on TV when the consumer might buy your competitor's product. When a specific breakfast cereal or soft drink is advertised, the vendor receives immediate profit from the effort. Who profits if a story about the remarkable healing benefits of intermittent fasting to reverse diabetes or obesity were featured on TV? Not the junk food industry. Not the pharmaceutical industry. You are only useful to this sickness management system if you are regularly consuming junk food and soft drinks and existing somewhere between well and dead. No one profits when you eat real food. Except you and your family.

Beta Carotene

When we take Mother Nature's wholesome food, we consume a rich mixture of known and unknown nutrients in synergistic combinations. There are over <u>300 studies showing that a diet rich in fruits and vegetables</u> lowers the risk for various cancers. [5] There are over 600 different carotenoids and 4000 unique bioflavonoids in whole fruits and vegetables, not to mention the various resistant starches (fiber) and vitamins, minerals, and potassium.

From this soup of anti-cancer substances, scientists randomly chose beta-carotene as their favorite ingredient, then created an all synthetic version (like the trans fat debacle mentioned before), coated the synthetic substances in coal tar derived coloring agents (known to be carcinogenic) and fed them to people who had been heavy smokers for decades. Didn't help. Might have increased the risk for lung cancer.[6] These synthetic pills were so far removed from whole fruits and vegetables that the study by the National Cancer Institute was laughable. Instead, doctors and the media warned patients about the hazards of beta carotene as a pill or in a food.

Sugar

Although sugar was first extracted from sugar cane in southeast Asia around 8000 BC, not until refining techniques were introduced and mass sugar cane plantations were planted around 1600 AD did the spread of sugar around the world commence. Yet sugar was expensive and only available in quantity to the gentile or royalty of the world. Thus began the diseases of civilization. Gout first became known as the rich 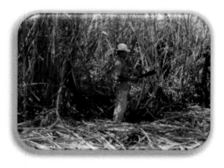 man's disease, because poor people never got gout.

The average American now consumes around 150 pounds/yr of refined sugar. In a study published in the Journal of the American Medical Association drinking too much sugary beverages causes 52,000 premature deaths annually in the US, while not eating enough fruit causes another 52,000 premature deaths.[7]

A roomful of PhDs from agribusiness have been trying to convince the public that the sugar in high fructose corn syrup, used liberally throughout the processed food supply, is the same as the fructose in fruit. Ignoring the fiber, potassium, thousands of phytochemicals, and alkalinizing effect of fruit; we are supposed to accept the propaganda that fruit and refined sugar are the same. Couldn't be further from the truth.

Sugarcane was the beginning of the "devil's triangle" which started with slave traders taking people from Africa to work the sugarcane fields in the Caribbean to bring sugar and its by-product rum to Europe. Everyone suffered in this multi-century tragedy.

Fruit and Health

While hundreds of studies have indicted refined sugar in a host of human ailments, not one study shows any deleterious effects from whole fruit. In a study done at Harvard, researchers followed 75,000 women for 24 years and found that 2 servings of peaches/week cut the risk of breast cancer by 40%.[8] See the chapter on "Foods with Anti-Cancer Activity" for more information on the healing power of whole fruit.

Whole Foods

Nature spends many millennia crafting and perfecting a food, then more millennia allowing humans to adjust to this food. Whole food contains:

- vitamins (known and yet to be identified)
- minerals (macro, micro and trace)
- minor dietary constituents (like lycopenes in tomatoes and ellagic acid in dark berries)
- conditionally essential nutrients (such as coenzyme Q in heart muscle and phytic acid in whole grains)
- fiber to feed our 100 trillion microorganism friends in our gut
- obscure substances that we are only beginning to study, such as phytoalexins in red and green fruits and vegetables

Whole food does not contain pesticides, herbicides, artificial coloring and flavoring agents, genetically modified organisms (GMO), antibiotics, veterinary drugs, and more.

Real food can work miracles in your body. The best studied diet on earth is the Mediterranean diet, which consists of a plant-based diet rich in fruits, vegetables, whole grains, legumes, nuts, seeds, and olive oil. Small amounts of fish and chicken are used, with red meat only a few times a month. This diet has been shown to reduce overall mortality by 60% when combined with light exercise, no smoking, and a few glasses of wine daily.[9] If the Mediterranean diet were a drug it would be publicized all over the media.

WHAT IS NOT IN WHOLE FOODS?

antibiotics
growth hormones
pesticides
herbicides
fungicides
hormone disrupters
toxic metals (i.e. arsenic)
aflatoxins (fungal by products)
etc.

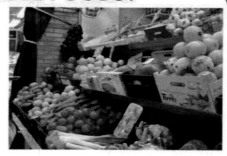

WHAT IS IN WHOLE FOODS?

Nature to be commanded must be obeyed.
Sir Francis Bacon (1561-1626) founder of scientific inquiry

"Look deep into nature and then you will understand everything better." Albert Einstein

Your Choice

You can choose to participate in the $1 trillion/yr junk food/tobacco/alcohol/soft drinks/fast food industry in America. If so, then you will be forced to participate in the $3.5 trillion/yr medical industrial complex, which includes the $440 billion pharmaceutical industry. Which all takes the posture "we are going to medicate the symptoms that occurred as the inevitable result of your unhealthy lifestyle." Or you can choose real food.

As demonstrated by Harvard physician and professor, John Abramson, MD, in his book <u>OVERDOSED AMERICA</u>: THE BROKEN PROMISE OF AMERICAN MEDICINE, food and lifestyle can prevent and reverse many common ailments in western society. Real food will give you real health. It's your call.

For more information about real food and healing go to GettingHealthier.com.

PATIENT PROFILE: Surviving asbestos cancer.

K.F. was diagnosed with mesothelioma, having spent some time in his youth working with asbestos. His original oncologist gave him an optimistic 6 months to live. He and his wife began using an aggressive diet and supplement program in conjunction with his chemotherapy. Three years later, K.F. still has the cancer, but has had an excellent quality of life, looks better than his neighbors, and has received a handsome legal settlement for his cancer from asbestos exposure. Once again, nutrition doesn't cure every cancer patient, but it usually provides a dramatic extension of quality and quantity of life.

ENDNOTES

[1] https://www.ncbi.nlm.nih.gov/pmc/articles/PMC6284174/
[2] https://www.ncbi.nlm.nih.gov/pmc/articles/PMC3742216/
[3] https://www.who.int/news-room/detail/14-05-2018-who-plan-to-eliminate-industrially-produced-trans-fatty-acids-from-global-food-supply
[4] https://onlinelibrary.wiley.com/doi/abs/10.1046/j.1365-2621.2002.00620.x
[5] https://www.tandfonline.com/doi/abs/10.1080/01635589209514201
[6] https://academic.oup.com/jnci/article/88/21/1550/928505
[7] https://jamanetwork.com/journals/jama/article-abstract/2608201
[8] https://www.ncbi.nlm.nih.gov/pmc/articles/PMC3641647/
[9] https://jamanetwork.com/journals/jama/article-abstract/199485

KEY 9
NUTRITION

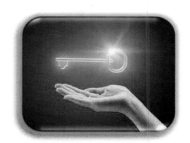

Chapter 9.4
Foods with Anti-Cancer Activity

"The western diet is fertilizer for cancer."
David Servan-Schreiber, MD, PhD
author of ANTI-CANCER: A NEW WAY OF LIFE

     Legumes, or beans, are an extraordinary health food. A 10 pound sack of dried beans will cost you around $10, becomes 30 pounds of cooked food, and last for months or years if kept properly. Beans can be sprouted to further enhance their nutritional value. When studying the Mediterranean diet, garbanzo beans (aka chickpeas) feature prominently as a staple.

     Garbanzo beans have been consumed for thousands of years in the middle east and can be pureed into hummus. Garbanzo beans are an excellent plant source of protein, rich in fiber, and capable of lowering appetite to enhance weight loss. In one study, equal amount of calories from garbanzo beans or bread were provided test subjects. The garbanzo beans <u>lowered insulin levels</u>, which is a major victory in health. Garbanzo and other beans have been shown to have **potent anti-cancer activity**.[1] Beans nourish the microbiome within your gut.

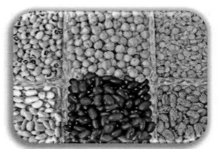

Eating more beans would not only improve the <u>health of the person, but the health of the planet</u>. Legume plants actually nourish the soil with nitrogenous organisms. It takes 2500 gallons of water, 12 pounds of grain, 35 pounds of topsoil, and the equivalent of one gallon of gasoline to produce one pound of beef. Start small with beans, if you are new to this game. Slowly build up your intake until your gut and your microbiome can digest the beans without flatulence. Chickpeas can be boiled, pressure cooked (preferred), or roasted and make a fabulous soup.

Not until the introduction of processed foods did cancer become a common cause of death. Yet even primitive healers noticed the link between diet and cancer. Chinese physicians 2000 years ago wrote: "an immoderate diet will lead to cancer." For most of the 20th century the authorities in government and medicine denied any link between nutrition and cancer. The problem has always been special interest groups. If the FDA, USDA, or AMA discourage the consumption of any food or group, that special interest lobby would assail the report and the people in charge. Which is why it took nearly a hundred years after smoking was known to be harmful before the Surgeon General issued his report in 1964 that smoking was probably not good for you.

In 1982 the National Academy of Sciences issued their report <u>DIET, NUTRITION, AND CANCER</u> [2] with the headlines "spread the good news, cancer may not be as inevitable as death and taxes." By

1991 the Office of Alternative Medicine issued a book NUTRITION IN CANCER TREATMENT which showed that nutrition (food and supplements) would assume a role as adjuvant therapies in cancer treatment. We are now 30 years beyond that report and most cancer patients are seriously mislead on the subject of nutrition.

The following are foods that have demonstrated anti-cancer activity, always to be used in conjunction with your doctor's best care. Recommendations are based on the best studied diet on the planet earth, the Mediterranean diet, which is plant based. There is irrefutable evidence that a plant-based diet (55-99% of kcal) is essential to prevent and reverse cancer. However, there are nutrients found in animal food that can be of benefit. When various scientists and explorers have studied diets throughout the world, there were no pure vegans anywhere. Some groups, including Seventh Day Adventists, have chosen to eat a vegan diet for religious reasons. Given the option, indigenous people throughout the world supplemented their plant-based diet with small amounts of clean wild caught animal food.

NUTRIENTS AS BIOLOGICAL RESPONSE MODIFIERS
changing the way the body works to reverse cancer

→IMMUNE REGULATORS, ELIMINATE INFECTIONS?
→ALTER GENETIC EXPRESSION OF CANCER
→CELL MEMBRANE DYNAMICS
→DETOXIFICATION
→PH MAINTENANCE, BALANCING PROTONS
→PROOXIDANTS & AOX, BALANCING ELECTRONS
→CELLULAR COMMUNICATIONS (signal cell transduction)
→PROSTAGLANDIN REGULATION
→STEROID HORMONE CONTROL
→ENERGY METABOLISM: AEROBIC VS ANAEROBIC
→PROBIOTICS VS DYSBIOSIS
→ANTI-PROLIFERATIVE AGENTS
→ALTER TUMOR PROTECTIVE MECHANISMS
→APOPTOSIS, PROGRAMMED CELL DEATH

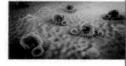

Choose often from the following group of plant foods:

FRUITS: apples, avocado, bananas, cantaloupe, etc.

VEGETABLES: asparagus, broccoli, carrots, cabbage, beets, pigmented potatoes, spinach, etc.

WHOLE GRAINS: amaranth, quinoa, barley, buckwheat, pigmented corn, brown rice, millet, oats, wheat* (unless you have gluten sensitivity)

LEGUMES: peas, beans, chickpeas, lentils, peanuts, etc.

NUTS: walnut, pecan, cashew, pine nut, Brazil nut, coconut

SEEDS: chia, hemp, papaya, poppy, sesame, pumpkin, watermelon, squash

SEAWEED/SEA VEGETABLES: kelp, kombu, wakame, nori, dulse, Irish moss

MUSHROOMS: shiitake, oyster, white button, maitake, Portobello, rei shi

MEDICINAL HERBS/HEALING SPICES: allspice, basil, bay leaf, celery seed, chili, clove, coriander, fennel, mint, mustard, horseradish, turmeric, oregano, sage, thyme, etc.

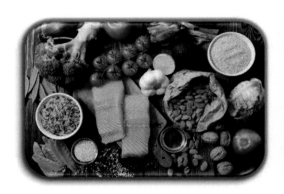

Choose occasionally from this group of animal foods:

POULTRY: chicken, turkey, eggs

FISH: salmon, sardine, trout, halibut, mahi, halibut, shrimp, lobster, oyster, clam

Chose rarely from this group of animal foods:

RED MEAT: grass fed beef, buffalo, goat

DAIRY: yogurt, cheese

Avoid

Hard liquor, hydrogenated fats, the whites (sugar, flour, potatoes, corn, rice), deep fried anything, GMO foods, fake foods

ORAC: OXYGEN RADICAL ABSORBENCE CAPACITY
sponges for free radicals

ORAC/5 GM	"...reduce risk of diseases of aging by adding high ORAC foods to diet." Floyd Horn, PhD, Tufts Univ.
prunes 288	
raisins 141	
blueberries 111	
blackberries 101	
garlic 96	*need 3000-5000 ORAC units/day*
kale 88	*(food & supplements)*
cranberries 87	*average US intake 1200 ORAC*
strawberries 76	
spinach raw 60	
plum 47	

Fruit

Fruit has been the ultimate health food, until the paleo and keto trends set in. For that reason, we are going to spend some time discussing the health merits of fruit. There is abundant misinformation that fruits are harmful since fruits contain natural sugars. While the Paleolithic and ketogenic diets have their place, they have eliminated or seriously reduced the most powerful anticancer food groups: fruit, whole grains, legumes. In fact, ALL scientific evidence shows that whole fruits are an important part of anyone's diet, especially the cancer patient. Whole fruits are a rich mixture of vitamins, minerals, bioflavonoids, carotenoids, pectin, fiber, potassium, and promising anti-cancer agents, such as ficin in figs and phytoalexins in red fruits. The antioxidant capacity (ORAC) and laxative effect of most fruits is therapeutic for the body.

Since sugar feeds cancer and fruits contain sugars, you might reason that whole fruit is ill advised for many people. Let's look at the evidence.

Does Fruit Increase Risk for Cancer?

In one study, Harvard researchers followed 75,000 women for 24 years and found that <u>2 servings of peaches per week lowered</u> the risk for breast cancer by 40%. [3]   If that was a drug, it would have been international headlines and peaches would be available only by prescription. In another study, Harvard researchers studied 44,000 men in Hawaii. The <u>more fruit they ate, the lower the risk</u> for cancer; in a dose dependent fashion. [4] Drug developers envy these kinds of results, then the press ignores it.

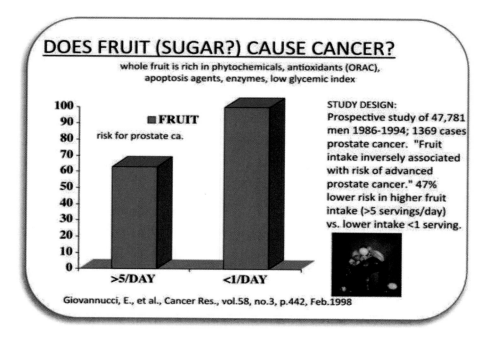

DOES FRUIT (SUGAR?) CAUSE CANCER?
whole fruit is rich in phytochemicals, antioxidants (ORAC), apoptosis agents, enzymes, low glycemic index

■ FRUIT
risk for prostate ca.

>5/DAY   <1/DAY

STUDY DESIGN: Prospective study of 47,781 men 1986-1994; 1369 cases prostate cancer. "Fruit intake inversely associated with risk of advanced prostate cancer." 47% lower risk in higher fruit intake (>5 servings/day) vs. lower intake <1 serving.

Giovannucci, E., et al., Cancer Res., vol.58, no.3, p.442, Feb.1998

Does Fruit Lower Immune Functions?

In a study of senior citizens in London, researchers found that the more whole fruit these people ate the lower the risk for shingles, a viral infection in the nerves. Those who ate less than one serving of fruit per week had a 300% increase in the risk for shingles compared to those who ate 3 servings of fruit per day.[5]

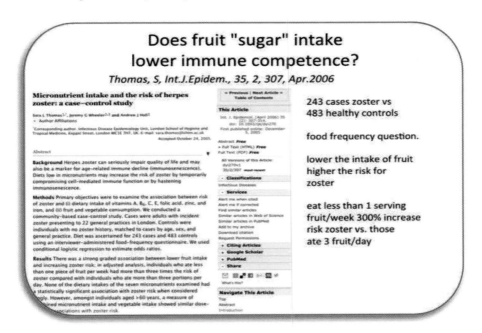

Does Fruit Promote Diabetes?

In a study examining 3.4 million patient years (patients x years followed) there was a significant decline in type 2 diabetes among those who ate more fruit, particularly grapes, apples, and blueberries.[6] However, fruit juice increased the risk for diabetes. Again, eat whole foods.

Fact is, fruit, eggs, and insects were the original caveman food, when intelligence and tools limited what was available to eat. Red and green fruits and vegetables contain phytoalexins, have powerful anti-cancer and anti-fungal activity. Here is where you begin to appreciate the brilliant design of nature. Fruit contains sugar, which fungus and insects would love to eat. Hence, fruits could only survive by producing substances that inhibit fungal growth, insects, etc. More than coincidentally, fungus and cancer can both be subdued by these anti-fungal compounds. Is cancer a fungal infection? More on that later.

BOTTOM LINE: Eat more fruit, especially organic, biodynamic, whole colorful fruit.

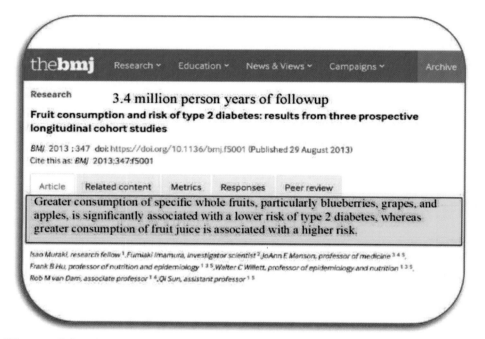

the**bmj**   Research ⌄   Education ⌄   News & Views ⌄   Campaigns ⌄   Archive

Research   **3.4 million person years of followup**
Fruit consumption and risk of type 2 diabetes: results from three prospective longitudinal cohort studies

BMJ 2013 ;347 doi: https://doi.org/10.1136/bmj.f5001 (Published 29 August 2013)
Cite this as: BMJ 2013;347:f5001

| Article | Related content | Metrics | Responses | Peer review |

Greater consumption of specific whole fruits, particularly blueberries, grapes, and apples, is significantly associated with a lower risk of type 2 diabetes, whereas greater consumption of fruit juice is associated with a higher risk.

Isao Muraki, research fellow [1], Fumiaki Imamura, investigator scientist [2], JoAnn E Manson, professor of medicine [3,4,5], Frank B Hu, professor of nutrition and epidemiology [1,3,5], Walter C Willett, professor of epidemiology and nutrition [1,3,5], Rob M van Dam, associate professor [1,4], Qi Sun, assistant professor [1,5]

Vegetables
This is a food group that receives nearly unanimous approval of nearly any doctor or health group. Asparagus, broccoli, carrots, cabbage, beets, pigmented potatoes, spinach, and more needs to be on your menu often. Try a green smoothie in your blender using spinach, peaches, and coconut milk. Try making roasted vegetables. Recipe is simple. Dice your favorite vegetables into a large blending bowl. Mix 1 cup of olive oil with small amounts of lemon juice, soy sauce, balsamic vinegar, and spices in abundance (see below) in a 2 cup container. Stir the liquid

ingredients, then spread over the bowl of mixed vegetables and mix thoroughly. Bake in 400 F oven for 30-40 minutes. Delicious.

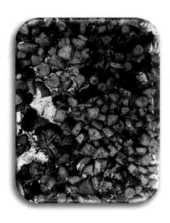

Whole Grains

Whole grains provided the basis for civilization. Our primitive ancestors were hunters and gatherers. They followed the herds. Yet, you cannot have a city until people settle down. It was in the Middle East that wheat was first cultivated, leading to farms, thus leading to cities, and specialization of labor. While the ketogenic and Paleolithic diet advocates have ruled whole grains as "unnecessary", nature and science say otherwise. The two longest ruling empires on earth, Egyptian and Roman, both made whole wheat their staple in the diet. The wheat we currently eat has been greatly modified in attempts to yield more gluten, which provide texture in making bread. Most modern wheat is genetically modified, then soaked in the herbicide glyphosate. Their wheat was different than our wheat. Yet, whole grains have provided humans with the bulk of calories and protein for centuries. Rice in Asia and South America. Quinoa among the Incas in South America. Corn among the Americas. Whole grains do not provide a complete protein, hence the need to add legumes and vegetables if you are seeking a vegan diet.

Whole grains provide more than just obvious nutrients, but also the prebiotics that your 100 trillion organisms in your gut require. Fiber from whole grains is fermented in the gut by bacteria to form by butyrate, which is essential for health of your gut lining. Early nutritionists identified fiber as indigestible, hence useless or counterproductive. Modern science finds that because fiber is indigestible it becomes essential for regularity and health of your gut microbiome.

Research shows that the more whole grains in the diet, the lower the risk. Beta glucans found in oats have shown tremendous health benefits,[7] including stabilizing blood glucose, improving serum lipids, upregulating the immune system through immunoglobulin and NK production. IP6 (inositol hexaphosphate 6) was once considered an anti-nutrient, or harmful, yet now shows promise as a <u>powerful anti-cancer agent</u>[8].

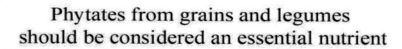

Phytates from grains and legumes should be considered an essential nutrient

International Journal of Food Science and Technology 2002, 37, 769–782

Anti-cancer function of phytic acid

Abulkalam M. Sham:

Department of Pathology.

Summary Inositol kingdo and its they a experin effects

Given the numerous health benefits, its participation in important intracellular biochemical pathways, normal physiological presence in our cells, tissues, plasma, urine, etc., the levels of which fluctuate with intake, epidemiological correlates of deficiency with disease and reversal of those conditions by adequate intake, and safety – all strongly suggest for its inclusion as an essential nutrient

Whole grains are best when steamed or pressure cooked. 3 cups of any whole grain with 6 cups of water in a pressure cooker for 15 minutes will yield a delightful part of your anti-cancer diet. Mix these whole grains with legumes and vegetables, or seafood, poultry and sea vegetables. Then have a party with the healing spices mentioned later.

Lectins merit special note here. There has been considerable interest in the PLANT PARADOX, which states that these commonly present lectins in plant food pose health hazards for humans. Lectins are carbohydrate binding proteins found in most plant food, particularly whole grains and legumes. The proponents of these theories recommend avoiding these foods, and/or selecting white rice over whole grain rice, and/or buying their pills to bind up the lectin in the gut.

Meanwhile, all of the data on lectins shows that they have no adverse effects in humans. In fact, <u>all of the data on the consumption of high lectin foods</u> (whole grains and legumes) actually shows that these foods lower the risk for heart disease, diabetes, cancer, and more.[9] Which is what you would expect with the brilliant designs in Nature.

Legumes

Having a sack of beans in the house is like having a roof over your stomach. Beans are an incredible addition to your anti-cancer diet. Dried beans will store for a year on the shelf, or many years in a vacuum sealed can. Great way to have food saved for a rainy day. Soybeans are a staple in Asia. Soy is an interesting food. Many studies have shown soy to be a valuable part of your anti-cancer diet. However, GMO soy (most of soy in America) is of less value. Genetically modified, then soaked in

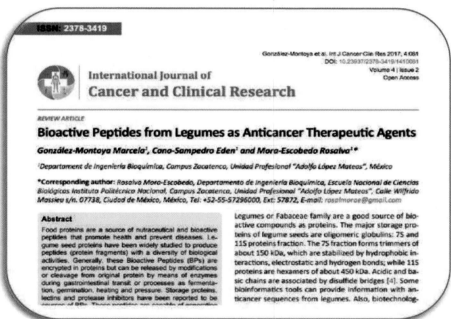

ISSN: 2378-3419

International Journal of
Cancer and Clinical Research

González-Montoya et al. Int J Cancer Clin Res 2017, 4:081
DOI: 10.23937/2378-3419/1410081
Volume 4 | Issue 2
Open Access

REVIEW ARTICLE

Bioactive Peptides from Legumes as Anticancer Therapeutic Agents

González-Montoya Marcela[1], Cano-Sampedro Eden[1] and Mora-Escobedo Rosalva[1]*

[1]Departamento de Ingeniería Bioquímica, Campus Zacatenco, Unidad Profesional "Adolfo López Mateos", México

*Corresponding author: Rosalva Mora-Escobedo, Departamento de Ingeniería Bioquímica, Escuela Nacional de Ciencias Biológicas Instituto Politécnico Nacional, Campus Zacatenco, Unidad Profesional "Adolfo López Mateos", Calle Wilfrido Massieu s/n. 07738, Ciudad de México, México, Tel: +52-55-57296000, Ext: 57872, E-mail: rosalmorae@gmail.com

Abstract

Food proteins are a source of nutraceutical and bioactive peptides that promote health and prevent diseases. Legume seed proteins have been widely studied to produce peptides (protein fragments) with a diversity of biological activities. Generally, these Bioactive Peptides (BPs) are encrypted in proteins but can be released by modifications or cleavage from original protein by means of enzymes during gastrointestinal transit or processes as fermentation, germination, heating and pressure. Storage proteins, lectins and protease inhibitors have been reported to be

Legumes or Fabaceae family are a good source of bioactive compounds as proteins. The major storage proteins of legume seeds are oligomeric globulins: 7S and 11S proteins fraction. The 7S fraction forms trimmers of about 150 kDa, which are stabilized by hydrophobic interactions, electrostatic and hydrogen bonds; while 11S proteins are hexamers of about 450 kDa. Acidic and basic chains are associated via disulfide bridges [4]. Some bioinformatics tools can provide information with anticancer sequences from legumes. Also, biotechnolog-

glyphosate, GMO soy and other GMO products should be avoided by most people and all cancer patients. The Paleo and ketogenic advocates often eliminate beans from the diet, under the assumption that beans may cause an adverse reaction, such as an auto-immune disease. Indeed, some people have adverse reactions to various foods. But in most cases, it is the person's gut that needs healing, not elimination of wholesome foods. More on the gut in the chapter on Microbiome.

The most scientifically examined and endorsed diet on earth, the Mediterranean diet, includes garbanzo beans often. Hummus is cooked garbanzo beans. In longevity studies, scientists find that the more beans people eat, the lower their risk for heart disease, cancer, diabetes, and nearly any other condition you can imagine. Beans are good for you.

Beans contain unique carbohydrates, stachyose and raffinose, that are of great interest to your gut bacteria, but must have a digestive enzyme in you to avoid gas and discomfort. To minimize flatulence from beans, soak them overnight, then discard the water, then pressure cook. Better yet, sprout the beans for 3-4 days, then pressure cook.

Beans contain anti-cancer substances [10] that have been researched and proven useful in your anti-cancer diet.

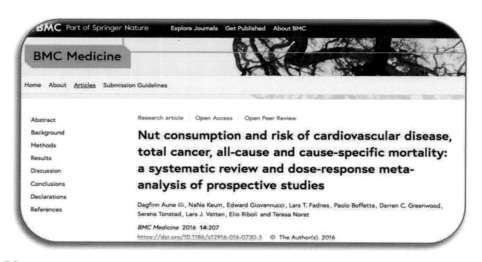

Nuts: Walnut, pecan, cashew, pine nut, Brazil nut, coconut

Consumption of nuts has consistently been shown to lower the risk for various diseases. For each 28 grams of nuts consumed (about a small handful) heart disease risk was lowered by 29%, cancer by 15%, death from lung problems 52%, infectious disease 75%, etc. The more nuts consumed, the better. Dose dependent response.[11]

Seeds: chia, hemp, papaya, poppy, sesame, pumpkin, watermelon, squash Seeds have the source of life within. Eat these foods often.

Seaweed: kelp, kombu, wakame, nori, dulse, Irish moss

Mar. Drugs **2014**, *12*(2), 851-870; https://doi.org/10.3390/md12020851   Open Access

Review

Fucoidan as a Marine Anticancer Agent in Preclinical Development

Jong-Young Kwak ✉

Department of Biochemistry, School of Medicine and Immune-Network Pioneer Research Center, Dong-A University, 32, Daesingongwon-ro, Seo-gu, Busan 602-714, Korea

Received: 15 November 2013; in revised form: 31 December 2013 / Accepted: 10 January 2014 / Published: 28 January 2014

Abstract: Fucoidan is a fucose-containing sulfated polysaccharide derived from brown seaweeds, crude extracts of which are commercially available as nutritional supplements. Recent studies have demonstrated antiproliferative, antiangiogenic, and anticancer properties of fucoidan *in vitro*. Accordingly, the anticancer effects of fucoidan have been shown to vary depending on its structure, while it can target multiple receptors or signaling molecules in various cell types, including tumor cells and immune cells. Low toxicity and the *in vitro* effects of fucoidan mentioned above make it a suitable agent for cancer prevention or treatment. However, preclinical development of natural marine products requires *in vivo* examination of purified compounds in animal tumor models. This review discusses the effects of systemic and local administration of fucoidan on tumor growth, angiogenesis, and immune reaction and whether *in vivo* and *in vitro* results are likely applicable to the development of fucoidan as a marine anticancer drug.

For much of human history, people living near the sea were a heartier group. There are many reasons for this advantage, including fish and kelp in the diet. There are hundreds of different land vegetables and hundreds of different sea vegetables (aka seaweed) categorized as either red, brown, or green. Green seaweed grows closer to the surface of the water, hence, the chlorophyll being used for photosynthesis. Red and brown seaweeds are found further below the water surface.

Over 2 billion people are deficient in iodine, with half suffering blatant iodine deficiency.[12] Seaweed solves this problem with therapeutic doses of iodine. From 33-68% of people in England and Germany have measurable problems with thyroid function due to iodine deficiency.

Seaweed is a rich source of most of the trace minerals required by the human body but not added to the soil in agribusiness. Fucoidan in seaweed is a <u>powerful anti-cancer substance</u>. [13] Several studies have shown a reduced risk for breast cancer with seaweed consumption.[14] 99% of the seaweed on earth is consumed in southeast Asia. Western palates are adapting to the rich flavor of seaweed. Some people say that dried kelp tastes like green potato chips.

Mushrooms: shiitake, oyster, white button, maitake, Portobello, reishi, lion's mane

There are many therapeutic benefits of edible mushrooms. <u>Maitake</u>,[15] shiitake, reishi, lentinan, and other mushrooms have been used for <u>centuries in Chinese medicine</u>.[16] Some mushrooms are capable of enhancing immune function to thwart infections and cancer. Culinary mushrooms are tasty and healthy. Medicinal mushrooms will be front line medicine of the 21st century.

Medicinal Spices

Grandmother was practicing herbal medicine all day everyday in the kitchen with her quiver of medicinal spices. Modern humans have substituted these powerful kitchen healers with salt, sugar, MSG, deep fried everything, and 2800 FDA approved food additives with questionable safety and no medicinal value. Columbus set sail over the edge of the earth in 1492 hoping to find a way to the "spice islands". In those days, food rotted quickly without the modern benefits of refrigeration or canning. Spices were used to cover the flavors of food that wasn't yet dangerous, but was not very fresh either. Spices were treasured by royalty and hoarded by peasants. We now know why. Spices not only improve the flavor of food but have extraordinary healing capacity. Scientists have proven beyond argument that medicinal spices could become front line therapies in the near future. Use these spices often liberally. For more details on the efficacy of these spices, see HEALING SPICES by Bharat B. Aggarwal, PhD.

Ajowan	Cumin	Pomegranate
Allspice	Curry leaf	Pumpkin seed
Almond	Fennel seed	Rosemary
Amchur	Fenugreek seed	Saffron
Aniseed	Galangal	Safe
Asafetida	Garlic	Sesame seed
Basil	Ginger	Star anise
Bay leaf	Horseradish	Sun-dried tomato
Black cumin seed	Juniper berry	Tamarind
Black pepper	Kokum	Thyme
Caraway	Lemongrass	Turmeric
Cardamom	Marjoram	Vanilla
Celery seed	Mint	Wasabi
Chile	Mustard seed	
Cinnamon	Nutmeg	
Clove	Onion	
Cocoa	Oregano	
Coconut	Parsley	
Coriander		

Putting It Together

Picture your plate as a clock face. Choose quality protein foods for one third of your plate. Choose cooked wholesome plant foods for the next one third of your plate. Choose raw colorful fresh fruits and vegetables for the last one third of your plate. You can do this.

EAT OFTEN

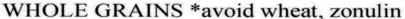

FRUITS
VEGETABLES
WHOLE GRAINS *avoid wheat, zonulin
LEGUMES
NUTS
SEEDS
SEA VEGETABLES
MUSHROOMS
MEDICINAL SPICES

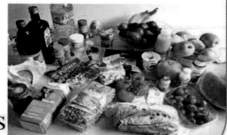

EAT OCCASIONALLY

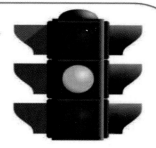

FISH
GRASS FED MEAT
EGGS
YOGURT
BUTTER

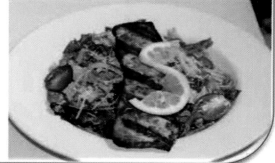

AVOID

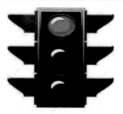

FAKE FOODS
WHITES: SUGAR, FLOUR, RICE, POTATO
DEEP FRIED ANYTHING
HYDROGENATED OILS
HARD LIQUOR

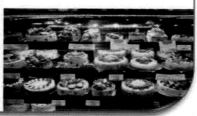

LOOKING AT A HEALTHY MEAL PLATE

tomato,spinach,carrot,peppers,
fruit,broccoli,cabbage,onion,etc

fish, wild game, poultry,
Grass fed beef, eggs,
beans, dairy,spirulina,kelp

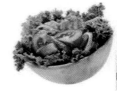

1/3
raw fr/veg

1/3
hi pro

1/3
cooked whole plant food

90% good
10% whatever

oatmeal,beans,rice,quinoa,tortilla,
yams,nuts,grains,legumes,cooked
vegetables, mushrooms, kelp

For more information about foods and their anti-cancer activity go to GettingHealthier.com.

PATIENT PROFILE: SHRINKING LUNG CANCER

C.G. was diagnosed with non-small cell lung cancer stage 3. The tumor was about the size of a tennis ball. C.G. began using the principles in this book along with chemo and radiation. Originally, his doctor gave him 6 months to live. That was 2 years ago. The tumor is now the size of a small marble and shrinking with each chest X ray and CT scan. Doctor said "I don't know what you are doing, but keep doing it." C.G. says "Thank you for writing your book. So far, you have saved my life."

ENDNOTES

[1] https://www.tandfonline.com/doi/abs/10.1080/01635581.2015.1004729
[2] https://www.nap.edu/catalog/371/diet-nutrition-and-cancer
[3] https://link.springer.com/article/10.1007/s10549-013-2484-3
[4] http://cancerres.aacrjournals.org/content/58/3/442
[5] https://academic.oup.com/ije/article/35/2/307/694696
[6] https://www.bmj.com/content/347/bmj.f5001
[7] https://onlinelibrary.wiley.com/doi/full/10.1111/j.1541-4337.2012.00189.x
[8] https://academic.oup.com/jn/article/133/11/3778S/4817990
[9] https://www.sciencedirect.com/science/article/pii/S0733521014000228
[10] https://www.tandfonline.com/doi/abs/10.1080/01635581.2015.1004729
[11] https://bmcmedicine.biomedcentral.com/articles/10.1186/s12916-016-0730-3
[12] https://www.ncbi.nlm.nih.gov/pmc/articles/PMC6284174/
[13] https://www.mdpi.com/1660-3397/12/2/851/htm
[14] https://www.ncbi.nlm.nih.gov/pmc/articles/PMC3651528/
[15] http://www.partnec.com/rd/rdgf/3/maitake_mxtract.pdf
[16] https://muse.jhu.edu/article/196008/summary

KEY 9
NUTRITION

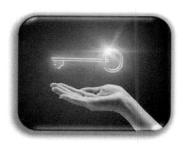

Chapter 9.5
Intermittent Fasting
Missing Link in True Health

"Why do they put lights in a refrigerator if you are not supposed to eat at night?" unknown

---

FROM NATURE'S PHARMACY: Blueberries

One of the more nutrient dense foods on earth, blueberries are low in calories but a treasure trove of antioxidants. As scientists unravel the mysteries of human health and our dance with our food supply, the subject of antioxidants has become quite common. Throughout nature there are free radicals, which are essentially electron thieves that destabilize molecules. Your immune system uses free radicals to douse invaders. Free radicals are a natural consequence of energy metabolism.

Chapter 9.5 – Intermittent Fasting. Missing link in true health

244

Pour some hydrogen peroxide on a piece of meat or spot of fresh blood and watch the bubbling of free radicals as they destroy the cell membrane of the blood or meat. Most experts agree that free radicals are a primary component to aging and cancer.

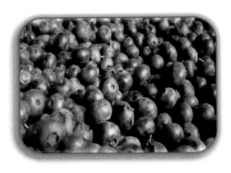

Antioxidants are electron donors, which quench the need for the free radical to destroy surrounding tissue. Many vitamins have antioxidant capacity, including C, E, beta-carotene. Flavonoids are particularly effective antioxidants and have opened a field of nutrition that holds great potential for preventing and reversing diseases. Anthocyanins from **blueberries directly increase** antioxidant capacity in humans.[1] Human subjects drank one liter of blueberry/apple juice daily for 4 weeks and demonstrated a **20% reduction in DNA damage**.[2] Blueberries help to prevent oxidation of the bad (LDL) cholesterol, help to prevent heart disease, prevent cognitive decline, and more. You may need to buy dried or frozen blueberries in order to get organic. Anytime you are eating the outside of the fruit or vegetable, it is worth pursuing organic. Blueberries: look great, taste great, and very healthy for your body. No downside here.

Inadvertent fasting has been with the human race since the dawn of time. We are built to fast. Our ancestors suffered through endless periods of fasting, famine, and other issues with their food supply. Humans have adapted to require frequent times of no food intake. Most religions include fasting as part of the annual rituals because it became obvious that fasting improves health. Then, along came the modern food supply with dehydration, freezing, refrigeration, and canning. Slice, dice, chop, and blend until the food has a shelf life of forever and is no longer recognizable as a real food. Fast no more. The feast is here. And so are the epidemic levels of disease.

White light is composed of the primary prism colors of red, orange, yellow, blue, indigo, and violet (ROY G. BIV). Take away any of those colors and you do not have white light. Same with healing. Your full spectrum healing program involves all of the keys mentioned in this book. This chapter is invaluable in rectifying many of the problems created through modern eating and lifestyle.

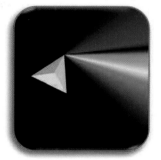

2/3 of Americans are overweight. Half of them are medically obese. We have TV shows to highlight "My 600 pound life" because there are so many "stars" in this category. The "Biggest Loser" TV show featured medically obese people who were given medical supervision for diet and exercise to lose weight. All of these people were given a caloric restriction program, meaning cut your calorie intake from 8000 per day as you are currently eating, to 1200 per day or less. There has never been a "class reunion" of the biggest loser winners (lost the most weight) because all of these people gained their weight back.

The domino of poor health starts like this. We eat. The body needs to digest that food and prepare for processing, receiving, and metabolizing the food. Insulin is secreted by the pancreas to allow glucose into the cells for the 100,000 chemical reactions that take place per second per cell. But the food intake is constant, just like the flow of insulin is constant, which creates insulin resistance on the cell membranes. The "noise" of constant eating, glucose, and insulin creates "deafness" or insulin resistance. So the body makes more insulin, which is an essential yet perilous hormone in the body. Excess insulin, such as is found in all type 2 diabetics and most Americans, causes weight gain, fat storage, inflammation, and a higher risk for cancer.

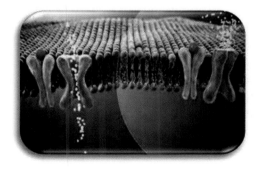

The benefits of fasting are extraordinary. Your humble author found out the easy way. I

Chapter 9.5 – Intermittent Fasting. Missing link in true health

246

practice what I preach. I live a healthy lifestyle. Am fit, trim, active. Yet for years my fasting blood glucose was in the 90-105 mg% range, which is pre-diabetic. HbA1C (glycosylated hemoglobin, a more accurate measure of chronic blood glucose) was 5.9, which is okay, but not great. Tried everything. Every diet, including Paleolithic and ketogenic, many different supplements. Nothing worked. Then I tried intermittent fasting (IF), by limiting my feeding "window" to 8 hours per day (e.g. eating from 10 am to 6 pm) and fasting one day a week. Within 3 weeks on this program my fasting blood glucose dropped to 67 mg% and I felt great.

Upon researching this subject, I found abundant data showing the **mental and physical benefits of IF**. For 2 million years of adaptation, humans faced chronic food scarcity. These cave dwellers were physically fit enough to catch and kill an animal or the human died. They consumed abundant plant food with naturally occurring pesticides that eventually became protective against aging and cancer. We now eat too much and too often. We are obese and unfit, and avoid any food that does not taste like ice cream or soda. And that lifestyle is killing advanced civilizations by the millions.

IF is being used by the best and brightest business people and athletes to **sharpen mental clarity** with "bio-hacking". IF has been shown to **lower the risk for** Alzheimer's disease, cognitive decline, and increase lifespan. IF gives the digestive tract a break, allowing for regeneration of cells. IF offers a **wealth of benefits** with zero cost. What does it cost to skip eating for 24 hours? Nothing. But since the biggest advertisers on TV are food and drugs companies who would all suffer revenue loss if broad portions of the population embraced IF, then you are not going to see articles on TV about this extremely important topic.

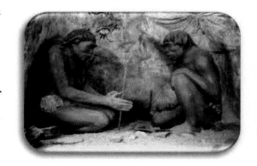

How Does it Work?

Think of your ancestors 20,000 years ago. Life was tough. Food supply was undependable. Predators were everywhere. If caveman and cavewoman went a week without food, then the adaptive forces of nature kicked in to generate a process of autophagy (auto=self, phagy=to eat). Your body begins this critical process of scavenging marginal cells to create newer, younger, faster, smarter cells. Nature is telling caveman, "you better get smart and fast enough to find food, or you are going to die." That is what IF does for us.

How Does it Help Cancer Patients?

Dietary restriction (DR) is the strategy of eating less calories, say dropping your intake from the necessary 2000 kcal/d to 1200 kcal/d, which eventually leads to some weight loss. But the long term benefits of DR have been mixed. There are a dozen good books for the public on the benefits of IF, starting with Jason Fung, MD <u>THE OBESITY CODE</u>. Dr. Fung is a diabetologist who found the treadmill of treating diabetics with renal failure discouraging. Upon research, Dr. Fung found that he could reverse/cure most type 2 diabetes with simple fasting.

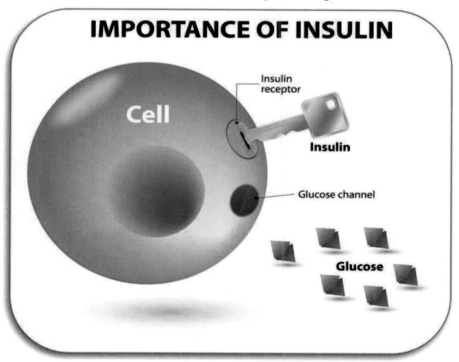

Chapter 9.5 – Intermittent Fasting. Missing link in true health

248

Meanwhile, <u>IF has been shown</u> to be a quick therapy to lower insulin like growth factor (IGF-1) which is a major accelerator of cancer growth. IF <u>enhances success rates</u> with chemo and radiation. Ketogenic and Paleolithic diets have their merits, but the inconvenient truth is that your body can generate glucose from protein, fat, or stored glycogen. By improving insulin sensitivity, you lower blood glucose and IGF…which is a major victory in your pursuit of wellness.

On the other hand, you cannot starve a parasite out of a host. You cannot starve a cancer out of the cancer patient. But you can make the cellular environment inhospitable for the cancer. Do not undertake excessive fasting without medical advice. Up to 40% of cancer patients actually <u>die from malnutrition</u>, which is due to the effects of cancer, many chemicals created by cancer cells, chemo and radiation, depression, and loss of appetite. Hence, the goal is to use strategic IF to make the body hostile toward cancer cells, while feeding the cancer patient adequate calories and protein to be able to maintain strength and host defense mechanisms.

What to Do?

Follow the dietary recommendations in this book on foods to eat. Take one day a week and eat no food, no calories, just water and tea. On the six days per week that you do eat, narrow your feeding "window" to 8 hours daily, such as from 10 am to 6 pm and eat enough to maintain optimal weight and strength. You not only are making it very uncomfortable for your cancer cells, but also rejuvenating your body and mind for the longer and smarter life that you will enjoy. On a risk to benefit to cost ratio, it doesn't get any better than IF.

For more information about intermittent fasting go to <u>GettingHealthier.com</u>

PATIENT PROFILE: SURVIVING KIDNEY CANCER

M.M. was diagnosed with renal cell carcinoma stage 4. She took thalidomide and interferon for nearly 2 years, then stopped these medications due to side effects, which included vomiting, headaches, and neuropathy (numb and painful hands and feet). M.M. used the nutrition guidelines in this book along with mistletoe and dendritic cell therapy to shrink her tumor by 30%. She was given 6 months to live, yet has survived 3 years, although she still has tumor burden. Her quality of life is good. M.M. says that "we are all terminal. Just try to make a difference in someone else's life."

ENDNOTES

1 https://www.ncbi.nlm.nih.gov/pubmed/12475297
2 https://www.ncbi.nlm.nih.gov/pubmed/17602170

KEY 9
NUTRITION

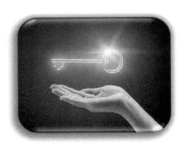

Chapter 9.6
Nutritional Supplements
for Optimal Health

"Individuals with special nutritional needs are not covered by the RDAs."
National Research Council, RECOMMENDED DIETARY ALLOWANCES, pgs1&8, Washington, 1989

FROM NATURE'S PHARMACY: Walnuts

Walnuts are the nutritional superstar among nuts. Walnuts contain healthy amounts of fiber, protein, antioxidants, and omega 3 (alpha linolenic acid) fats. Most Americans do not get enough omega 3, which is also found in oily fish like salmon. **Each gram of omega 3 fat per day** lowers risk of heart disease by 20%.[1] Although nuts are high in calories and fat, nut eaters are more likely to be lean and non-diabetic. Other nuts include peanut (actually a legume), pistachio, pine nut, almond, pecan, chestnut, macadamia. In a meta-analysis of 7 huge studies covering 3.7 million subject years (people x years studied), researchers found nut consumption significantly reduced the **risk for heart disease and cancer.**[2] Lightly roast walnuts or pecans in a 400 F oven for about 10 minutes. Delicious!

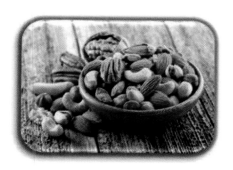

This chapter alone could have been a thousand-page tome. You have been spared the daunting task of searching through the quagmire of facts about nutrition supplements and cancer. Supplements are not a cure for cancer. But supplements can provide a tremendous boost to your body's quest to heal itself. This chapter summarizes the risk to benefit to cost ratio of nutrition supplements and makes recommendations for what to do.

While Big Pharma claims that the $37 billion/yr supplement industry is unregulated, that is not true. FDA maintains control over the manufacturing and advertising of nutrition supplements. The problem is that there are no deaths from nutrition supplement usage, in spite of the fact that 68% of Americans take supplements and 84% express satisfaction with the safety and outcome of their supplement usage. Meanwhile, 55% of Americans take some prescription drug as part of this $448 billion year empire where at least **128,000 people die from the on label use of the drugs.**[3] Nutrition supplements, when the right nutrient at the right dosage is chosen, can contribute significantly to making the body self-regulating and self-repairing.

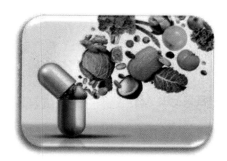

This chapter is designed to be a primer on nutrition supplements for cancer patients undergoing medical therapy. Much more details can be found in the reference texts listed below. In every aspect of life there is a wide gap between surviving and thriving. There are at least one billion people around the world at the very brink of death from starvation. 2 billion are deficient in iodine. 500,000 children go blind annually for lack of vitamin A. Surviving but not thriving. Babies have survived being thrown into dumpsters. Not a good start to life and certainly not an optimal situation. Nutrition supplements can bring a person beyond surviving into thriving.

According to extensive research from the United States Department of Agriculture 92% of Americans DO NOT GET the Recommended Dietary Allowance (RDA, now called Reference Daily Intake, or RDI) for all listed essential nutrients. And there is compelling evidence that the RDA is a survival level for nutrient intake, not a level that allows for optimal health, nor recovery from cancer.

There are now over 20,000 scientific references that support the use of supplementing a good diet with vitamins, minerals, herbs, fatty acids, glandular extracts, probiotics, and food extracts.

For more information see:
BEATING CANCER WITH NUTRITION, by Patrick Quillin, PhD,RD,CNS
PDR FOR NUTRITIONAL SUPPLEMENTS, by Sheldon Hendler, MD, PhD
NUTRITIONAL MEDICINE, by Alan Gaby, MD
DISEASE PREVENTION AND TREATMENT, Life Extension Media
ENCYCLOPEDIA NATURAL MEDICINE, Murray, ND & Pizzorno, ND
NUTRITIONAL INFLUENCES ON ILLNESS by Melvyn Werbach, MD

Look at the label for dog and cat food. The ingredients are loaded with added vitamins and minerals because everyone wants "Fluffy" to be healthy. Note the list of trace minerals found in expensive plant fertilizers. None of these products are sold due to the "placebo" effect, or simply because the animal or plant believed in the product. Nutrients, like drugs, have a dose-dependent response curve. Meaning, the more you give, the greater the effect, until additional benefits taper off and toxicity becomes possible.

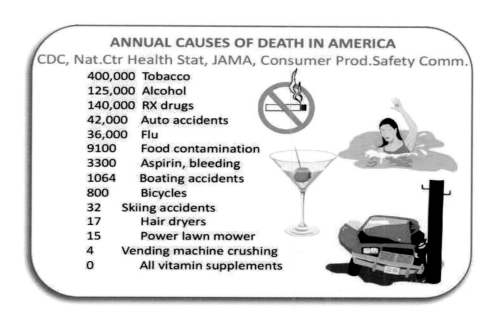

ANNUAL CAUSES OF DEATH IN AMERICA
CDC, Nat.Ctr Health Stat, JAMA, Consumer Prod.Safety Comm.

400,000	Tobacco
125,000	Alcohol
140,000	RX drugs
42,000	Auto accidents
36,000	Flu
9100	Food contamination
3300	Aspirin, bleeding
1064	Boating accidents
800	Bicycles
32	Skiing accidents
17	Hair dryers
15	Power lawn mower
4	Vending machine crushing
0	All vitamin supplements

Reasons to Consider Taking Nutrition Supplements

1. Not eating an ideal diet. Which is most of us.
2. Our soil is not properly fertilized with minerals, leaving the food we eat with <u>much less minerals</u> than our ancestors. [4]   Minerals like magnesium, selenium, boron, chromium, vanadium, lithium and more are extremely important in human biochemistry, yet rarely added to the soil in fertilizer. Our ancestors added wood ash to soil for a decent effort at providing mineral content in the food supply.
3. Toxin exposure. While people living in clean environments can exist on lower doses of some nutrients, exposure to toxins increases the need for many nutrients to protect us from the diseases and metabolic wrecking balls from thousands of poisons in our environment.
4. Stress. <u>Stress increases the need for many nutrients</u> while lowering the absorption of nutrients through changes in peristalsis, secretion of digestive enzymes and leaky gut. [5]
5. Beyond deficiencies. For most of the 20th century, nutrition scientists focused on observing frank clinical deficiency syndromes: scurvy for

vitamin C, beriberi for thiamin, pellagra for niacin, etc. Yet researchers now find an abundance of data showing that marginal intake of nutrients can lead to fragile DNA which leads to cancer or premature aging. There is a wide gap between surviving and thriving when it comes to nutritional intake.

6. Nutrients as biological response modifiers. Nutrients are Mother Nature's version of wonder drugs. Fish oil and lithium can improve mental functions. Various antioxidants can slow the oxidation that induces aging and cancer. Various nutrients can slow down the glycation, or cooking our tissues from too much blood sugar. Most Americans are deficient in magnesium, which has a <u>powerful anti-cancer effect</u>.[6] Humans have been exposed to these nutrition factors for eons, which makes these nutrition supplements vastly more safe than patented pharmaceuticals that are foreign to the human body. Nutrients are unpatentable, yet extremely potent, cheap and safe ways to improve bodily functions.

Risks of Nutrition Therapy

In an extensive review of the literature found in the New York Academy of Sciences textbook BEYOND DEFICIENCIES (vol.669, p.300, 1992), Dr. Adrienne Bendich found the following data on nutrient toxicity:

ï B-6 can be used safely for years at up to 500 mg (250 times RDA)

ï Niacin (as nicotinic acid) has been recommended by the National Institute of Health for lowering cholesterol at doses of 3,000-6,000 mg/day (150-300 times RDA). Time-release niacin is more suspect of causing toxicity as liver damage.

ï Vitamin C was tested in 8 published studies using double-blind placebo-controlled design. At 10,000 mg/day for years, vitamin C produced no side effects.

ï High doses of vitamin A (500, 000 iu daily) can have acute reversible effects. Teratogenicity (birth defects) is a possible complication of high dose vitamin A intake.

ï Vitamin E intake at up to 3,000 mg/day (300 times RDA) for prolonged periods has been shown safe.

ï Beta-carotene has been administered for extended periods in humans at doses up to 180 mg (300,000 iu or 60 times RDA) with no side effects nor elevated serum vitamin A levels.

In MICRONUTRIENTS AND IMMUNE FUNCTION (NYAS, vol.587, p.257, 1990), John Hathcock, PhD, a Food and Drug Administration toxicologist, reported the following data on nutrient toxicity:

ï Vitamin A toxicity may start as low as 25,000 iu/day (5 times RDA) in people with impaired liver function via drugs, hepatitis, or protein malnutrition. Otherwise, toxicity for A begins at several hundred thousand iu/day.

ï Beta-carotene given at 180 mg/day (300,000 iu or 60 times RDA) for extended periods produced no toxicity, but mild carotenemia (orange pigmentation of skin).

ï Vitamin E at 300 iu/day (30 times RDA) can trigger nausea, fatigue, and headaches in sensitive individuals. Otherwise, few side effects are seen at up to 3,200 iu/day (320 times RDA).

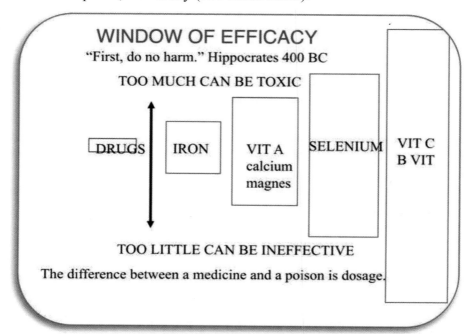

WINDOW OF EFFICACY

"First, do no harm." Hippocrates 400 BC

TOO MUCH CAN BE TOXIC

DRUGS   IRON   VIT A   SELENIUM   VIT C
               calcium   B VIT
               magnes

TOO LITTLE CAN BE INEFFECTIVE

The difference between a medicine and a poison is dosage.

ï   B-6 may induce a reversible sensory neuropathy at doses of as low as 300 mg/day in some sensitive individuals. Toxic threshold usually begins at 2,000 mg for most individuals.

ï   Vitamin C may induce mild and transient gastro-intestinal distress in some sensitive individuals at doses of 1,000 mg (16 times RDA). Otherwise, toxicity is very rare at even high doses of vitamin C intake.

ï   Zinc supplements at 300 mg (20 times RDA) have been found to impair immune functions and serum lipid profile.

ï   Iron intake at 100 mg/day (6 times RDA) will cause iron storage disease in 80% of population. The "window of efficacy" on iron is probably more narrow than with other nutrients.

ï   Selenium can be toxic at 1-5 mg/kg body weight intake. This would equate to 65 mg/day for the average adult, which is 812 times the RDA of 80 mcg. Some sensitive individuals may develop toxicity at 1,000 mcg/day.

Synergism of Nutrients

Then we get to the fascinating subject of synergism, or the combined effect is greater than the sum of the parts…e.g. $1 + 1 = 3$ or 500. Imagine a home construction site where all the necessary supplies are delivered in the right ratio: lumber, drywall, nails, concrete, electrical wiring, plumbing pipes, etc. The workers build the house in very efficient fashion. But what happens if one or more of those building materials is short changed or not delivered at all? Big problems in the construction process. Same with nutrients being delivered to your body. When your body receives the optimal amounts of nutrients and in the proper ratio, then true magical healing can occur.

In a study conducted on female rats, researchers gave the animals various combinations of nutrients while exposing the rats to DMBA (one of the carcinogens in tobacco smoke). The animals that got DMBA all died. The animals that got DMBA but were also provided with nutrition supplements of EITHER selenium, or magnesium, or vitamin C, or vitamin A all had a roughly 50% reduction in mortality from cancer. The next group of animals were given the DMBA plus a combination of 2 nutrients: either selenium plus vitamin A, or magnesium plus vitamin C, or vitamins A plus C. In this group there was a roughly 70% reduction in

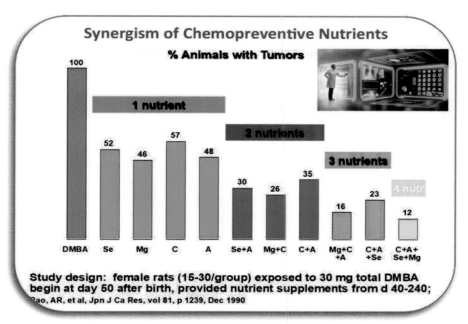

Synergism of Chemopreventive Nutrients

% Animals with Tumors

Study design: female rats (15-30/group) exposed to 30 mg total DMBA begin at day 50 after birth, provided nutrient supplements from d 40-240; Rao, AR, et al, Jpn J Ca Res, vol 81, p 1239, Dec 1990

death. The next group of animals received 3 nutrients: either magnesium plus C plus A, or C plus A plus selenium. This group had a roughly 80% reduction in mortality. The final group of animals were exposed to the DMBA then received four nutrients: C plus A plus selenium plus magnesium. This group had an 88% reduction in mortality. The more nutrients that are added to the equation, the better the outcome. The point is: you want nutritional synergism working for you to produce optimal health, especially while fighting cancer

Choosing Your Vitamin Supplements

There are hundreds of vitamins, minerals, botanicals (herbs), fatty acids, food extracts, glandular extracts, probiotics, prebiotics, mushroom extracts, seaweed extracts and other nutrient compounds that can be of benefit to the medically treated cancer patient. None are cure alls. You can do your own scavenger hunt among these options, or you may wish to investigate "one-stop shopping" options:

Suggested Nutrition Supplements for the Medically Treated Cancer Patient

VITAMINS

Vitamin A (As Beta Carotene)
Vitamin A (As Palmitate)
Vitamin C (As Ascorbyl Palmitate)
Vitamin D (As Cholecalciferol)
Vitamin E (As Tocopheryl Succinate)
Vitamin E (As Mixed Tocopherols)
Vitamin K1 (As Phytonadione)
Thiamine
Riboflavin
Niacin (Nicatinic Acid)
Niacinamide
Vitamin B6 (as Pyridoxine HCl)
Vitamin B6 (as P5P)
Folate (as L-5-Methylfolate, glucosamine salt)
Vitamin B12 (As Methylcobalamin)
Biotin
Pantothenic Acid
Vitamin K2 (As Menaquinone-7)

MINERALS

Calcium D-Glucarate
Potassium Iodide
Magnesium
Zinc Glycinate
L-Selenomethionine
Manganese Glycinate
Chromium Polynicotinate
Molybdenum
Potassium
Vanadyl Sulfate
Lithium Orotate
Boron

CONDITIONALLY ESSENTIAL NUTRIENTS

Choline Bitartrate
Inositol
Alpha Lipoic Acid
L-Carnosine
CoQ10
Pterostilbene
RNA
N-Acetyl-L-Cysteine (NAC)

PHYTONUTRIENTS

Bioflavonoid Complex	Green Tea
Inositol Hexaphosphate 6	Boswellia
Pine Bark, Ellagic Acid	Bioperine
Resveratrol	Beet Root
Turmeric Extract BCM-95	Spirulina
Blueberry Concentrate	Citrus Pectin
Broccoli Powder (TrueBroc)	Jiaogulan

AMINO ACIDS

Bovine Tracheal Cartilage
L-Lysine
L-Proline
L-Glycine

MUSHROOMS

Cordyceps Extract
(Cordyceps sinensis)
Maitake D Fraction
Shitake

SEAWEED

Fucoidan

1) Inexpensive, easy, one scoop of powder per day mixed in your green smoothie drink or applesauce, 40 ingredients ImmunoPower Light found at ImmunoPower.com/light

2) Premium and comprehensive, one scoop of powder per day mixed in your green smoothie drink, 70+ ingredients ImmunoPower 7.0 Bundle with Antarctic Krill Oil found at ImmunoPower.com

Working with your doctor, choose the supplement regimen that best suits your ability to tolerate vitamins and your ability to pay for them.

For more information on the efficacy of nutrition supplements for improving outcome for medically treated cancer patients, see the chapter "Nutrition is Essential in Cancer Treatment".

For more information about nutrition supplements go to GettingHealthier.com.

PATIENT PROFILE: BEAT TERMINAL BREAST CANCER

Y.K. was diagnosed with inflammatory stage 4 breast cancer and given 6 months to live. Y.K. knew that medical therapy probably couldn't cure her cancer. She asked her oncologist about nutrition as helpful or adjuvant therapy along with the chemo and radiation that had been proposed. Her oncologist said "no nutrients". So Y.K. changed oncologists. Her new oncologist accepted, but did not encourage, the use of nutrients during chemo. Y.K. used an aggressive combination of foods and supplements that she learned about in BEATING CANCER WITH NUTRITION to help put her terminal breast cancer into remission within a year, and she remained disease-free five years later, at which point your author lost contact with her. Y.K. told me that she "had to slow down and lose my perfectionism" once she got the cancer diagnosis. Her words of encouragement to you, dear reader, is "Life is worth living. We need to treat our body with respect or we won't have life." As an interesting footnote to Y.K.'s cancer, her dog developed breast cancer. Even after chemo, the dog continued to deteriorate. Y.K. gave her dog nutrition supplements and mistletoe injections subcutaneously, which put her dog into remission. Both Y.K. and all of her dogs are doing well at last report.

ENDNOTES

[1] https://www.ncbi.nlm.nih.gov/pubmed/23076616
[2] https://academic.oup.com/ajcn/article/101/4/783/4564522
[3] https://health.usnews.com/health-news/patient-advice/articles/2016-09-27/the-danger-in-taking-prescribed-medications
[4] https://www.scientificamerican.com/article/soil-depletion-and-nutrition-loss/
[5] https://psychologyofeating.com/4-ways-stress-impacts-digestion/
[6] https://www.sciencedirect.com/science/article/abs/pii/0306987780900109

KEY 9
NUTRITION

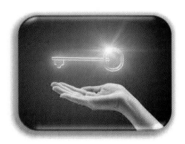

Chapter 9.7
Recipes

PLANNING YOUR MEALS

Eating should be both nourishing and fun. Of the hundreds of dietary programs that have been studied, none has been more thoroughly endorsed by the scientific community than the Mediterranean diet. This sample meal plan outlines the typical foods you eat under the Mediterranean diet. It covers the three main meals per day for a whole week. Keep in mind that this is just a rough guide to help you get started.

Some people have adverse food reactions. If you can't eat that food, then delete it. Feel free to add and remove items to fit your individual needs. While the scientific evidence overwhelmingly supports a plant based diet, there is mixed reviews on strict vegan diet. Two days here are vegan. Other days offer small servings of chicken, grass fed beef, fish, eggs, yogurt, and cheese.

This diet will be a dramatic improvement over the Standard American Diet (SAD). This diet offers you the taste, cost, convenience, nutrition, and health that you both like and deserve.

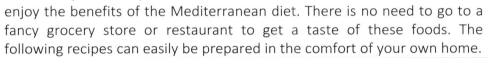

The serving portions are variable. This is to encourage you to adjust your servings and eating habits according to your own needs. It is up to you to make sure that you are not eating too much at any time.

This chapter contains a few useful recipes for anyone who wants to enjoy the benefits of the Mediterranean diet. There is no need to go to a fancy grocery store or restaurant to get a taste of these foods. The following recipes can easily be prepared in the comfort of your own home.

Potatoes: Pigmented are welcome. Purple, yams, sweet
Beverages: Teas, coffee, coconut milk, homemade nut milk, filtered water, red wine at dinner
Oatmeal: From rolled oats
Sweeteners: Honey, stevia, dried fruit
Meats and butters: Grass fed
Abundant use of medicinal spices: turmeric, cinnamon, pepper, ginger, rosemary, cumin, cardamom and others
Electric pressure cooker to prepare beetroot and brown rice.

Bonus Recipes

The end of this chapter contains several bonus recipes you can exchange as you wish.

Day 1

- Breakfast
  - o Frittata with Broccoli and Fresh Herbs
  - o Tomato-Cucumber Relish
  - o Fresh grapefruit
  - o Mango Celery Smoothie
- Lunch
  - o Hemp Tabouli Salad
  - o Fresh Asparagus Soup with Vegetable Broth
- Snack
  - o Broiled Tomatoes on Toast
- Dinner
  - o Fish with Tomato-Caper Sauce
- Desert
  - o Lemony Cheesecake with Mixed Berry Jam

Day 2 - Vegetarian

- Breakfast
  - o Nut Butter with Banana and Chia Seeds
  - o 1 cup Greek yogurt. Honey OK if needed
  - o Kale, Cucumber & Apple Smoothie
- Lunch
  - o Easy Ratatouille
  - o 1 cup of red grapes
- Snack
  - o 6 to 12 whole almonds
- Dinner
  - o Vegetable Patties with Coriander & Cloves
  - o Selection seasonal vegetables
- Dessert
  - o Orange-Banana Muffins

Day 3

- Breakfast
  - Broiled Tomatoes with Parmesan Cheese
  - Mint Watermelon Smoothie
- Lunch
  - Falafel with Condiment of Your Choice
  - Ginger Sesame Spinach Salad
- Snack
  - Baby carrots with 1 to 2 tbsp of hummus tahini
- Dinner
  - Chicken with Red Wine
  - Steamed vegetables of your choice
- Dessert
  - Dark Chocolate Peanut Butter Cups

Day 4

- Breakfast
  - Quinoa Fruit with Black Beans
  - Greek Yogurt
  - Carrot Juice
- Lunch
  - Gazpacho
  - 1-2 slices of gluten-free toast
- Snack
  - ½ piece of whole-grain pita pocket and 1 tbsp of tapenade
- Dinner
  - Beef & Vegetable Stew – Pressure Cooker
  - Steamed broccoli, hot Pepper flakes, olive oil
- Dessert
  - Vegan Layer Bar with Salted Caramel Sauce

Day 5

- Breakfast
    - o Sweet Potato and Black Bean Burrito
    - o ½ cup Greek yogurt with prune puree or fresh berries
    - o Purple Power Pick Me Up Smoothie
- Lunch
    - o Macedonian Salad
    - o ½ cup fresh pineapple chunks
- Snack
    - o 1 cup organic popcorn
- Dinner
    - o Mediterranean Citrus Chicken
    - o Fresh seasonal vegetables of your choice
- Dessert
    - o Fudge with Lentils

Day 6 - Vegetarian

- Breakfast
    - o Almond Couscous
    - o Greek yogurt
    - o Savory Tomato Juice
- Lunch
    - o Creamy Mustard Salad
    - o Eggplant Dip on Toast
- Snacks
    - o Broccoli florets dipped in olive oil lemon juice
- Dinner
    - o Herb Roasted Mediterranean Vegetables
    - o Slices of apple dipped in 1 tbsp of almond butter
- Dessert
    - o Ricotta with Honey and Almonds

Day 7

- Breakfast
  - o Vegetable Couscous with Curry
  - o Ginger Turmeric Smoothie
- Lunch
  - o Grilled Chicken or Seafood
  - o Greek Salad
- Snacks
  - o 2 fresh apricots or other small fruit and ½ cup yogurt or cottage cheese
- Dinner
  - o Indian Chickpeas in a Bowl
- Dessert
  - o Chocolate Avocado Pudding with Sea Salt

Day 1

Breakfast

Frittata with Broccoli and Fresh Herbs

Servings: 4-6   Prep: 15 mins   Cook: 15 mins

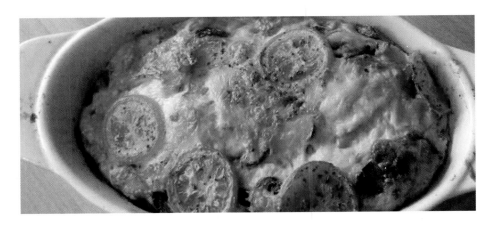

12 med-large organic eggs
1 pepper, chopped
1 medium red onion, chopped
12 oz broccoli florets, finely
chopped
1 tomatoes, chopped
2 cloves garlic, crushed

2 cups spinach, chopped
¼ cup fresh parsley, chopped
1 tbsp Italian herbs
1 tsp salt and pepper to taste
1 tbsp olive oil
4 oz Parmesan cheese, grated

Optional: See Condiment Section at end of chapter

Directions

1. In a 10 inch oven safe frying pan (you will be baking later), sauté onion in olive oil to an almost done. Remove onion and set aside.
2. On medium high heat toss in chopped peppers, broccoli and garlic. Add additional olive oil if needed.
3. In a separate bowl, use a fork to whisk the eggs.
4. Add remaining ingredients: spinach, parsley, herbs, salt, pepper.
5. Heat oven to 350 degrees.
6. Pour egg mixture into pan and stir. Sprinkle with Parmesan.
7. Place in the oven - bake for 15 minutes. Let cool for 5-10 minutes prior to serving.

Variation Suggestions:
Asparagus and Goat Cheese: Omit broccoli and add 1 pound asparagus, trimmed and cut into ¼ lengths, lemon zest and juice. Add goat cheese in Step 6.
Mushroom and Pecorino Frittata: Omit broccoli and substitute 1 pound cremini mushrooms, stemmed and cut into ½ inch pieces. Add ¼ cup green scallions and ¼ cup Pecorino Romano in Step 6.

SMOOTHIE - Mango and Celery
Servings – 4   Prep – 10 mins   Cook – 0 mins

2-3 leaves of kale
1 ¼ cups frozen mango
2 celery stalks

2 oranges, juiced
¼ cup flat-leaf parsley
¼ cup fresh mint

Directions
Place all ingredients in high speed blender until liquid. Serve over ice.

Lunch

Hemp Tabouli Salad
Servings: 2   Prep: 10 mins   Cooking: 0 mins

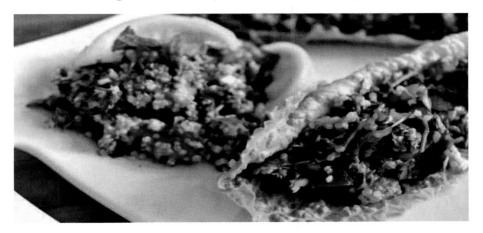

½ cup parsley, fresh
½ cup mint leaves, fresh
1/8 tsp sea salt
2 medium tomatoes
1 cup shelled hemp seeds

2 tbsp coconut water
½ lemon, juiced
¼ cup hemp oil
1 lettuce head

Directions:
1. Finely chop and combine parsley, mint, and sea salt.
2. Transfer herbs and salt to a large mixing bowl.
3. Add tomatoes, hemp seeds, oil and coconut water.
4. Mix well, and serve with fresh lettuce.
5. Store remaining in refrigerator for up to 2 days

Fresh Asparagus Soup with Vegetable Broth
Servings: 2   Prep: 15 mins   Cook: 0 min

1 pound fresh asparagus
¾ cup onion, chopped
½ cup vegetable broth
1 tbsp butter
2 tbsp arrowroot
1 cup nut milk
Pinch ground black pepper
1¼ cups vegetable broth
½ cup Greek yogurt
1 tsp lemon juice

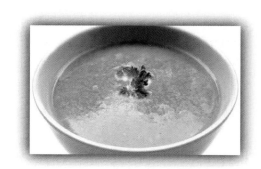

Directions
1. Place asparagus and onion in a saucepan with ½ cup vegetable broth and arrowroot.
2. Bring the broth to a boil, reduce heat and let simmer until vegetables are tender. Reserve a few asparagus tips for garnish.
3. Blend remaining vegetable mixture and puree until smooth.
4. Melt butter in the pan that was used for asparagus and onions. Add salt and pepper to the butter, stir. Cook mixture for only 2 minutes.
5. Stir in remaining 1 ¼ cups vegetable broth and increase the heat.
6. Continue stirring until mixture simmers.
7. Stir the vegetable puree and milk into the saucepan.
8. Whisk yogurt into the mixture.
9. Stir until heated. Add lemon juice. Ladle into individual bowls
10. Garnish with reserved asparagus tips. Salt as needed.

Dinner

Fish with Tomato-Caper Sauce

Servings – 4   Prep – 20 mins   Cook – 30 mins

4 pieces of grilled or broiled
salmon, salmon, cod, mahi,
shrimp, sardines
2 pieces tomatoes, large seeded
and chopped

1 clove garlic, minced
¼ cup capers
1 tsp dried tarragon
1 tsp extra virgin olive oil
Black pepper and sea salt to taste

Directions

1. Combine the tomatoes, garlic, capers, tarragon, pepper, salt, oil.
2. Spoon over the seafood.

Dessert

LEMONY Cheesecake with Mixed Berry Jam

Servings – 8   Prep – 30 mins   Cook – 60 mins

Base:
1 ½ cups oats,
  lightly toasted
1 cup dates, pitted
½ cup cashews
6 tbsp butter or coconut oil,
  melted
½ tsp cinnamon
¼ tsp salt

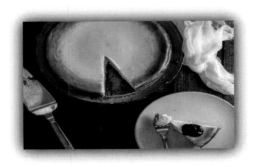

Filling:
2 large eggs
2 ⅓ cups cottage cheese
1 cup Greek yogurt
⅓ cup honey

2 tbsp lemon juice
2 tsp vanilla
2 tsp arrowroot
Toppings: 2 cups mixed berries

Directions

1. Line bottom of 8-inch spring form with parchment paper. Oil the sides of the pan. Preheat oven to 350 degrees.
2. *Crust.* In a food processor, grind the oats into flour, add dates and cashews. Add melted butter OR coconut oil, cinnamon and salt. The dough should be crumbly. If dates were a little dry, add approx. 1 tbsp of warm water and blend quickly on low.
3. Gently press the crust into lined pan. Set aside.
4. *Filling.* Blend filling ingredients: on low speed; cottage cheese, yogurt, honey, lemon juice, vanilla, arrowroot until smooth.
5. Beat eggs separately, add to Filling mixture. Mix well.
6. Pour everything into the pan. Bake in the oven for about 1 hour.
7. *Mixed Berry Jam.* Process berries, strain to remove excess water
8. Chill then garnish with fresh whipped cream and mixed berry jam. Finely chopped pecans can also be added.

Day 2 - Vegetarian

Breakfast

Nut Butter with Banana and Chia Seeds
Servings – 2   Prep – 5 mins   Cook – 0 mins

2 slices gluten free bread, toasted
1 small banana
1 tbsp chia seeds

1-2 tbsp nut butter
(almond, peanut, cashew)

Directions

Spread nut butter on toast, add sliced banana, and sprinkle with chia seeds.

SMOOTHIE – Kale, Cucumber & Apple
Servings – 2   Prep – 5 mins   Cook – 0 mins

4 leaves of kale	1 cup grapes, seedless
2 cucumbers	½ lemon, peeled, no seeds
2 apples	½ inch ginger root, grated
4 celery stalks	Water as needed

Directions:
Place all ingredients in a high speed blender. Serve with ice immediately.

Lunch

Easy Ratatouille
Servings – 4   Prep – 20 mins   Cook – 35 mins

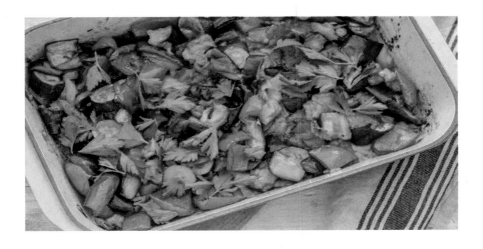

1 tbsp olive oil
2 large onion, chopped
4 large tomatoes
2 large bell peppers, chopped
2 large eggplants, diced
6 oz mushrooms, chopped
4 large zucchini, diced

1 8 oz can tomato paste
3 cloves garlic, minced
2 tbsp dried basil
¼ cup fresh parsley
¼ cup fresh dill
Salt and pepper to taste

Directions

1. Heat olive oil in a large saucepan over medium-high heat. Add onion, tomatoes, bell peppers and sauté 5 minutes.
2. Add eggplant and mushrooms, cover and cook 5 minutes.
3. Stir in zucchini, tomato paste, garlic and basil. Simmer gently 20 mins.
4. Stir in parsley, dill, salt and pepper. Cook 5 minutes more, stirring occasionally.
5. Serve garnished with chopped parsley and dill.

Dinner

Vegetable Patties with Coriander& Cloves

Servings – 4 to 6   Prep – 20 mins   Cook – 35 mins

Ground Paste Ingredients:
2 tbsp grated coconut
4 green chili peppers, finely chopped
1 small onion, chopped

4 cloves garlic, chopped
1 tsp cloves
1 stick fresh cinnamon
2 tsp coriander leaves, chopped
Salt to taste

Patties:
2 tbsp olive oil
4 onions, finely chopped
½ cups green peas parboiled
2 potatoes, boiled, chopped fine
2 cups vegetables (cauliflower, beans, carrots) chopped finely

2 small beetroot boiled, chopped
1 tbsp lemon juice
2 tbsp coriander leaves, chopped
2 tbsp butter
Salt to taste

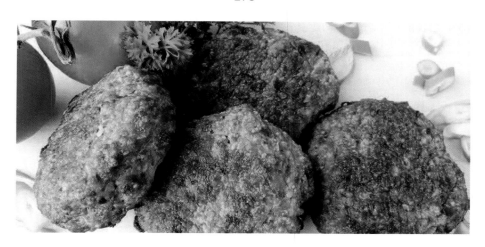

Directions

1. *Ground Paste*: Heat the oil in a pan, sauté onions on medium heat for about 3 minutes. Add ground paste ingredients and stir for about 2 minutes or till aromatic.
2. *Patties*: Add chopped mixed vegetables and green peas. Sauté on high heat for 2-3 mins, until vegetables are well coated with the paste. Cover and cook on low heat. Continue stirring every few minutes until half cooked.
3. Add boiled potato and beetroot. Sprinkle with salt to taste. Mix well. Cover and cook on low heat, stirring every few minutes.
4. Add lemon juice and chopped fresh coriander leaves.
5. Shape the mixture into patties.
6. Heat griddle and add 1 tbsp butter. Place 4-5 patties on the griddle and brown each side (drizzle oil as needed while turning) golden brown. Cook remaining patties.

Dessert

Orange-Banana Muffins
Servings – 12   Prep – 20 mins   Cook – 20 mins

3 cups rolled oats
½ cup of almonds
1 tbsp of baking powder
1 egg
1 cup orange slices, blended
1 ripe banana, mashed

1 cup applesauce, unsweetened
½ cup pumpkin puree
 (canned is ok)
¼ cup plain Greek yogurt
¼ cup honey (adjust to taste)
1 tbsp of vanilla

Directions
1. Preheat your oven to 375 degrees
2. Combine oats and almonds using a blender to grind to flour. Pour into a large mixing bowl. Stir in baking powder. Beat the egg in another bowl and add the oranges, banana, applesauce, and pumpkin.
3. Stir vanilla and honey into yogurt
4. Add 1/3 of the oat mixture to the banana mixture and stir until combined. Add half of the yogurt. Sir until combined.
5. Continue with the rest of the oats, yogurt and banana mixture.
6. Use olive oil cooking spray on 12 muffin cups then fill with batter.
7. Bake for 20 minutes or until the middle sets. Remove from oven and cool for 15 minutes then remove from the muffin tin. Cool before serving.

Day 3

Breakfast

Broiled Tomatoes with Parmesan Cheese
Servings – 6   Prep – 20 mins   Cook – 70 mins

6 medium fresh tomatoes
2 tbsp fresh basil, chopped
 or 2 tsp of dried basil

2 tbsp Parmesan cheese, grated
2 tbsp of extra virgin olive oil
½ tsp salt to taste

Directions

1. Core tomatoes and cut them in half.
2. Heat olive oil in a skillet over a medium heat until the aroma is released (5 mins).
3. Put the tomatoes cut side down and cook until crispy for another 5 minutes. Turn and add a sprinkle of salt, cheese, basil.
4. Broil tomatoes until the cheese melts and the tomato is slightly browned.

SMOOTHIE – Mint Watermelon
Servings – 2   Prep – 5 mins   Cook – 0 mins

¼ watermelon
½ cup nut milk

1 lime, juiced
4 leaves mint, finely chopped

Directions

Place all ingredients in a high speed blender. Blend with ice if desired.

Lunch

Falafel with Condiment of Your Choice
Servings – 4 to 6   Prep – 20 mins   Cook – 40 mins

15-oz can garbanzo beans
2 cloves garlic, mined
1 medium onion, chopped
1 large egg, lightly beaten
1 cup almonds or other nut, ground
1 tsp dried oregano

½ tsp ground cumin
1 tbsp lemon juice, fresh
Olive oil cooking spray
Pepper and salt to taste

Directions

1. Process the garbanzo beans, garlic, onion, cumin and oregano in a food processor.

2. Season with lemon juice, pepper and salt; stir in ½ ground almonds or nuts and egg
3. Spread remaining ground nuts on a plate. Make 16 round balls from the bean mixture; roll them on ground almonds for coating. Set these balls on wax paper.
4. Spray a large skillet with your olive oil cooking spray. When the skillet is hot, add falafel balls to cook until browned, about 10 minutes.
5. Serve with condiment of your choice,

Optional: See Condiment Section at end of chapter

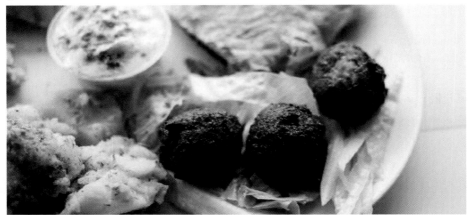

Ginger Sesame Spinach Salad
Servings – 2 to 4   Prep – 15 mins   Cook – 60 mins

Salad

2 chicken breasts,
  cooked (optional)
3 cups spinach
1 avocado, cubed

1 carrot, chopped
1 tbsp cilantro, roughly chopped
¼ cup onion, thinly sliced
1 tsp sesame seeds

Ginger Sesame Dressing
¼ cup olive oil

½ red pepper, seeded, chopped

½ lime, juiced
1 tbsp coconut milk or water
½ inch ginger root, grated

1 tbsp apple cider vinegar
1 clove garlic
¼ tsp toasted sesame oil

Directions
1. Place all salad ingredients in a large bowl.
2. Mix all dressing ingredients in a blender until smooth. Pour dressing over salad. Salt as needed.

Dinner

Chicken with Red Wine
Servings – 4 to 6   Prep – 20 mins   Cook – 60 mins

1 chicken, cut up
¼ cup of red wine
¼ cup of red wine vinegar
½ cup of pitted ripe olives
3 cloves of minced garlic
1 orange, juiced

¼ cup of extra virgin olive oil
1 tbsp oregano leaves, dried
1 tsp paprika
2 tbsp fresh parsley, chopped
¼ cup honey, as needed

Directions
1. Mix in vinegar, oil, olives, garlic, orange. Pour this mixture on the chicken in a resealable plastic bag.
2. Marinade chicken in the refrigerator for 2 hours. Turn occasionally.
3. Put the chicken in a shallow baking dish and add honey.
4. Pour wine into the pan and cook at 350 degrees for an hour or until thoroughly cooked. Basting every 20 minutes.
5. Sprinkle parsley, oregano and paprika before serving.

Dessert

Dark Chocolate Peanut Butter Cups
Servings – 2-4   Prep – 15 mins   Cook – 35 mins

16 oz dark chocolate chopped
  (at least 60% cacao)
½ cup nut butter (peanut,
almond, pecan or other)
3 tbsp coconut oil

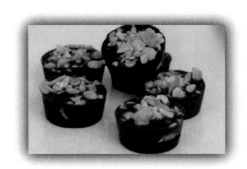

Directions
1. Melt the chocolate, use either a double boiler or a large bowl placed over, but not touching, a pot of boiling water.
2. In a small bowl, combine the peanut butter with the remaining 1 tbsp. coconut oil.
3. Line a plate or muffin pan, with cupcake liners. I recommend using stronger liners for the extra support.
4. Pour the melted chocolate mixture to cover the bottom of each liner.
5. Allow to set in the freezer for about 5 minutes.
6. Once set, add a small scoop of the peanut butter mixture into the center of the cup. Flatten with your thumb or the back of a spoon.
7. Pour additional melted chocolate over the peanut butter to cover, about 1-2 tbsps.
8. Place back into the freezer for about 25-30 minutes to completely set.

Day 4

Breakfast

Quinoa with Black Beans

Servings – 2-4   Prep – 15 mins   Cook – 0 mins

1 cup cooked quinoa
  (try tricolor)
1½ cup black beans, cooked
½ cup tomato, deseeded
½ cup shallots
1 mango, diced

Honey Lime Glaze:
¼ cup honey
2 tbsp lime juice
1 tbsp basil or parsley, garnish

Directions
1. Allow quinoa to cool to room temperature.
2. In a large bowl, combine quinoa, black beans, tomato, shallots, and mango.
3. *Glaze*: In a small bowl combine honey and lime juice. Drizzle over quinoa and toss.
4. Garnish with chopped fresh basil and/or parsley

Carrot Juice

Servings – 2-4   Prep – 10 mins   Cook – 0 mins

8 carrots
2 apples
¼ tsp cinnamon
1 large head of romaine lettuce
1 cup water

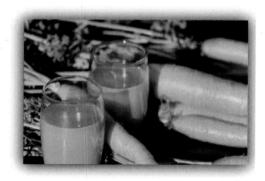

Directions
Place all ingredients in a high speed blender.

Lunch

Gazpacho
Servings – 4   Prep – 15 mins   Cook – 0 mins

4 tomatoes, seeded, chopped
2 cloves of minced garlic
½ cup bell peppers, chopped
½ cup cucumber,
  peeled and chopped
½ cup red onion, chopped

¼ cup of extra virgin olive oil
¼ tsp ground cumin
1 lemon, juice
1 cup vegetable broth
4-6 ice cubes
Dash of cayenne pepper

Directions
1. Using a blender, mix all ingredients until smooth.
2. Chill mixture for at least 2 hours or overnight.
3. Serve with gluten free bread

Dinner

Beef & Vegetable Stew with Pressure Cooker
Servings – 6   Prep – 10 mins   Cook – 30 mins

A great dish to make the day before to allow the flavors to mix.
Perfect to freeze.

2 tbsp olive oil,
  plus extra to drizzle
2 lb grass fed beef
6 oz tomato paste
1 medium onion, finely sliced
1 carrot, chopped
1 celery stick, chopped
2 colored potatoes, chopped

4 large garlic cloves, chopped
4 cups beef broth
Pinch ground cloves
A few fresh thyme sprigs
¼ cup parsley
2 tbsp ghee or butter
Salt and pepper to taste

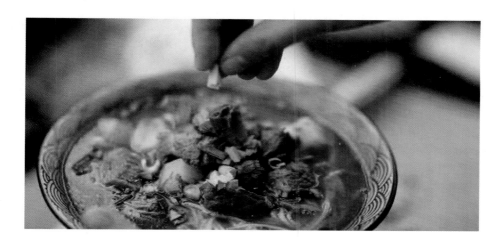

Directions

1. Heat the ghee on sauté. Brown the beef for 7-8 mins. Add onions, garlic and keep stirring for 5 mins.
2. Add remaining ingredients and seal. Cook on high for 10 minutes. Do a quick release.
3. Serve with steamed broccoli drizzled with hot pepper flakes and olive oil.
4. Cover and refrigerate the stew for up to 5 days or freeze. Reheat gently in a low oven or on the stovetop over low heat.

Optional: rice noodles can be added if desired.

Dessert

Vegan Layer Bar with Salted Caramel Sauce

Servings – 8   Prep – 20 mins   Cook – 50 mins

Almond Crust
1½ cups almond flour (or chickpea,
cassava, coconut or hazelnut flour)
2 ½ tbsp pure honey
1/3 cup coconut oil, softened

Vegan Layer Bars
1/2 cup mixed nuts, chopped
¾ cup dark chocolate chips
½ cup coconut flakes, unsweetened
½ cup almonds, chopped

Salted Caramel Sauce:
¼ cup coconut oil
¼ cup pure honey
2 tbsps almond butter
¼ tsp pure vanilla extract
⅛ tsp sea salt

Condensed Coconut Milk:
1 13.5 oz. can coconut milk
1/3 cup pure honey

Directions

1. Preheat oven to 350 degrees F. Line baking dish with parchment paper, set aside.
5. *First layer*: almond crust. In a large bowl, add almond flour, honey, softened coconut oil. Mix to create a dough that holds together when pressed.
6. Press this dough evenly into the bottom of a baking dish.
7. Bake until it's slightly browned, about 14-16 mins. Remove from oven
8. *Second layer:* Sprinkle chopped mixed nuts over top. Lightly press the nuts into the almond meal crust.
9. Add coconut flakes and dark chocolate chips on top.
10. *Salted caramel sauce.* In a saucepan on medium heat, combine coconut oil and honey. Stir. Heat thoroughly, then add almond butter, whisk together until smooth.
11. Remove from heat; add vanilla extract and sea salt.
12. Drizzle salted caramel sauce over the layer of dark chocolate chips. Then top with chopped almonds.

13. *Condensed coconut milk.* In a saucepan on medium heat whisk coconut milk and honey. Bring mixture to a low boil, stirring frequently. Reduce to a simmer for 15-20 minutes, stirring frequently. The sauce will reduce by half.
14. Remove the sauce from the heat and allow to slightly cool.
15. Pour 1 cup sweetened coconut milk evenly over the top of the bars. Allow the mixture to be absorbed through layers.
16. Place baking dish in oven and bake until sides are lightly golden brown, and the top is melted. About 30 minutes.
17. Remove from oven and cool. Chill and slice into squares.

Day 5

Breakfast

Sweet Potato and Black Bean Burrito
Servings – 6   Prep – 15 mins   Cook – 15 mins

These burritos are freezer-friendly. Wrap in plastic wrap, then in foil and place in freezer. To reheat, remove foil and plastic/ Place in oven on 350 degrees for 15 mins.

6 (8-inch) whole wheat tortillas
3 medium sweet potatoes
1 15 oz can black beans
¼ tsp cumin
¼ tsp chili powder
Few dashes of red pepper flakes
6 large eggs

1 avocado, diced
½ cup mozzarella cheese, shredded
1/3 cup red enchilada sauce
1 cup Greek yogurt or salsa
1 ½ tbsp ghee

Directions
1. Cook sweet potatoes until soft. Mash with a fork, set aside.
2. In a separate large bowl, add black beans, cumin, chili powder and red pepper flakes if desired. Stir to combine then set aside.

3. In a separate medium bowl, beat eggs. Add 1 ½ tbsp ghee to pan and cook eggs. Fold every few minutes for fluffy eggs. Once cooked, remove from heat.
4. To assemble burritos, warm tortillas (It makes them easier to roll) and lay out, then evenly spread mashed sweet potato on each.
5. Spread scrambled eggs, diced avocado, black beans, and cheese on each tortilla.
6. Drizzle tbsp of enchilada sauce in each. Season with salt and pepper, if desired.
7. Tuck ends in, roll up burritos.
8. To warm: Place on baking sheet in oven at 300 degrees for 5-10 minutes.
9. Serve with Greek yogurt, salsa, or hot sauce.

Smoothie - Purple Power Pick Me Up
Servings – 2-3   Prep – 10 mins   Cook – 0 min

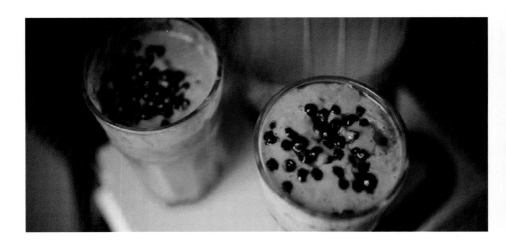

2-3 leaves of chard
1 beet, finely chopped
1 orange
1 cup strawberries or other berry

1 lime, juiced
½ inch ginger root, grated
½ inch of turmeric, grated
½ cup water, as needed

Directions

Place all ingredients in a high speed blender.

Lunch

Macedonian Salad

Servings – 4   Prep – 20 mins   Cook – 0 min

1 lemon
1 cup seedless grapes
1 cup halved strawberries
1 cup melon cubes or balls
1 cup peaches, cubed
1 cup mixed nuts
½ cup of red wine
Honey or stevia to taste

Directions

1. Roll the lemon on the counter, cut into quarters then set aside.
2. Gently combine remaining fruits in a large bowl and squeeze the lemon quarters over them. Avoid breaking the fruit.
3. Pour a little honey and drizzle with wine, then toss gently.
4. Let it stand at room temperature for 10 to 15 minutes then serve.

Dinner

Mediterranean Citrus Chicken

Servings – 4   Prep – 30 mins   Cook – 50 mins

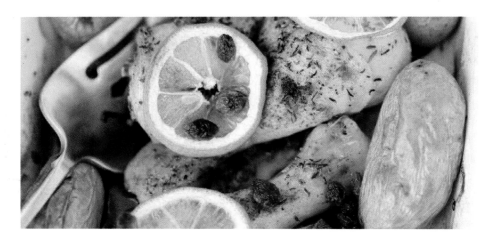

4 chicken breast halves, sliced
2 cups fresh greens
1 tsp olive oil
1 tsp arrowroot
1 tsp water
1 tbsp honey
¼ cup of chicken broth

½ cup juice and zest from
  orange, lemon, lime
1 orange (for garnish)
Sprigs of Italian parsley
  (for garnish)
1 tbsp ghee

Directions

1. Combine half the citrus juices and zest in resealable bag. Add the chicken
2. Seal the bag and lay it on a baking pan. Turn it over several times making sure that the chicken is covered well.
3. Place this in the refrigerator and marinade for at least 2 hours or overnight. Store the rest of the zest and juice in an airtight bowl.

4. Put chicken broth and olive oil in a skillet with ghee on a high heat until it simmers. Add the chicken without the marinade and reduce heat to medium.
5. Cook the chicken until the pink disappears for about 20 to 25 minutes. Turn halfway.
6. Combine other half juice and zest in a separate saucepan. Warm for 5 mins.
7. Make a paste with the arrowroot and water. Whisk this with the juice mixture and stir constantly until mixture thickens, about 20 minutes remove from heat.
8. Cover your platter with fresh greens and place the chicken over these. Drizzle with remaining sauce and add remaining zest.
9. Arrange slices of orange and parsley sprigs for garnish.

Dessert

Fudge with Lentils

Servings – 16-20 pieces   Prep – 45 mins   Cook – 20 mins

3.5 oz split lentils
16 oz water
2 cups nut milk
½ cup coconut flakes, unsweetened
10 almonds, chopped
2 tbsp pistachios, chopped
1 tsp cardamom powder
½ cup ghee
1/3 cup honey
 (more can be added)

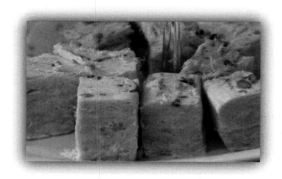

Directions

1. Soak the chickpeas in the water set aside 2-3 hours.
2. Strain chickpeas and cook in 1 cup milk till soft. Keep aside.
3. Blend the chickpea mixture to a coarse paste.

4. Heat ghee in a saucepan, add the chickpea paste.
   Cook until light brown.
5. Add honey and blend into the mixture.
6. Add remaining milk. Cook till the mixture leaves the sides of the pan.
7. Add the coconut flakes, almonds, pistachios and cardamom. Mix well
8. Remove from heat and spread onto a greased tray.
9. Cool and slice.

Day 6 - Vegetarian

Breakfast

Almond Couscous

Servings – 4   Prep – 10 mins   Cook – 0 mins   Stand – 2 hours

This recipe can be made ahead of time.
Let stand for the fresh flavors to blend.

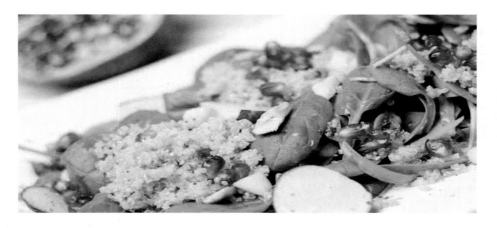

2 cups dry couscous
4 cups of water
½ cup of raisins or sultanas
½ cup almonds, chopped
½ cup pomegranate seeds

  or chopped grapes
2 radishes
1 tsp each ginger, cinnamon
  and cumin
4 cups spinach

Dash salt, black pepper
Red pepper to taste

1 tbsp of olive oil

Directions
1. Place couscous in a bowl and add boiling water. Cover immediately.
2. Let stand for 5 minutes or until all the liquid is absorbed.
3. Stir almonds, spices, raisins/ sultanas. Then olive oil after it is thoroughly combined.
4. Let stand at room temperature for 2 hours while flavors combine.
5. Serve on bed of spinach. Garnish with radish,
6. Refrigerate leftovers and serve the next day for the best-tasting breakfast.

Savory Tomato Juice
Servings – 2   Prep – 20 mins   Cook Time – 0 mins

4 tomatoes
2 carrots
1 celery stalk

1 radish
2 limes, peeled
1 dash of salt

Directions
Place all ingredients in high speed blender. Serve over ice and drink right away.

Lunch

Creamy Mustard Salad

Servings – 4   Prep – 20 mins   Cook Time – 0 mins

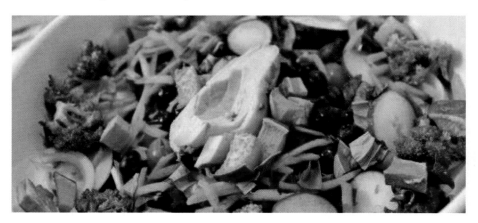

1 head of lettuce	½ cucumber
1 small head broccoli, lightly steamed	½ cup onion, sliced
	1 cup cherry tomatoes
1 large yam, colored	2 carrots, shredded

Optional: See Condiment Section at end of chapter for Mustard Dressing

Directions

1. Preheat oven to 375°F. Wash and chop yam into small cubes (if using).
2. Line baking sheet with parchment and place sweet potatoes flat on the baking sheet. Bake for 30-40 minutes.
3. Start steaming your broccoli.
4. While the yams cook, chop lettuce, cucumber, onion and tomatoes, shred carrot. Then add to a large bowl along with cooked broccoli.
5. *Dressing.* See mustard dressing below

Eggplant Dip on Toast

Servings – 6   Prep – 15 mins   Cook – 70 mins

Very similar to ratatouille, however the difference is the taste. Eggplant dip is served at room temperature and has a very robust taste. Used as a spread, dip or on toast.

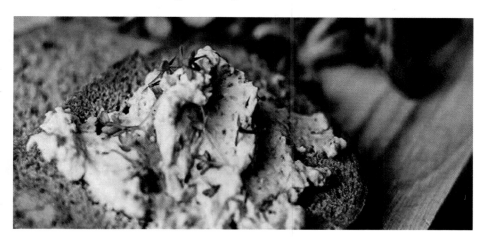

1 medium eggplant
1 tbsp sea salt
1 medium red bell pepper, chopped
1 medium yellow bell pepper, chopped
½ tsp red pepper flakes
1 tbsp honey

1 tbsp red wine vinegar
1 cup black olives, pitted, chopped
1 tbsp fresh basil, chopped
1 tbsp fresh parsley, chopped
¼ cup of capers, rinsed, drained
2 cloves of garlic, minced

Serving Suggestions:
Spread on gluten free toast
Vegetables for Dipping: Carrots, cucumbers, celery, or other seasonal vegetables

Directions

1. Cut the eggplant into cubes and put in colander and toss with sea salt. Cover with towel and leave on sink. Drain for 30 minutes.
2. Spray olive oil cooking spray on skillet and heat over medium-high heat. Rinse and dry eggplant and cook in skillet.
3. Reduce heat to medium-low and add onion, garlic and olive oil. Sauté for about 15 minutes until onion is soft.
4. Add bell peppers, red pepper flakes, honey and vinegar and cook or about 30 minutes. Continue simmering for another 30 minutes or until well cooked.
5. Add olives, basil, parsley, and capers and stir thoroughly. Remove from heat and let it stand to cool down.
6. Serve immediately or store in an airtight container.

Dinner

Herb-Roasted Mediterranean Vegetables
Servings – 4 to 6   Prep – 20 mins   Cook – 40 mins

8 cups root vegetables, assorted, chopped. (Suggest yams, carrots, parsnips, purple potatoes, sweet potatoes)	2 tsp parsley, chopped
	2 tsp rosemary, chopped
	1 tsp basil, chopped
1 large red onion	Salt and black pepper to taste
2 cloves garlic, minced	¼ cup of extra virgin olive oil

Directions

1. Toss the vegetables together with herbs, garlic, oil, salt and pepper. Place in a shallow pan.
2. Bake at 375 degrees in the oven for 40 minutes or until vegetables become tender. Stir once or twice during cooking.

Dessert

Ricotta with Honey and Almonds

Servings – 4 to 6   Prep – 20 mins   Cook – 30 mins

1 cup whole milk ricotta	1 tsp honey
½ cup almonds, sliced	Zest from an orange, optional
¼ tsp almond extract	Fruit, optional

Directions
1. Combine ricotta, almonds and almond extract in a bowl. Stir and combine.
2. Spoon into large or individual serving bowls.
3. Sprinkle with sliced almonds. Drizzle honey.
4. Serve with seasonal fruit.

Day 7

Breakfast

Vegetable Couscous with Curry

Servings – 4 to 6   Prep – 20 mins   Cook – 30 mins

1 cup couscous, cooked	2 tbsps of extra virgin olive oil
2 cups vegetable broth	½ cup parsley and chives
1 cup zucchini, chopped	2 tsp curry powder (turmeric,
½ cup carrots, grated	chili powder, coriander, cumin,
1 medium red onion, chopped	ginger)
2 tomatoes, seeded and chopped	1 tsp red pepper flakes
1 clove garlic, minced	Salt and pepper to taste

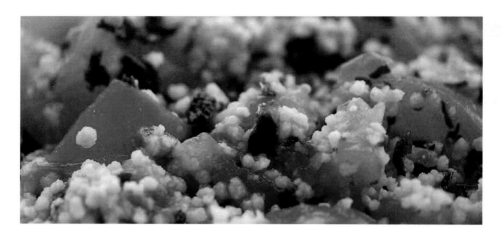

Directions
1. Bring broth to a boil and stir in couscous. Remove from the heat.
2. Let couscous stand covered for 5 minutes.
3. Heat a large skillet and add zucchini, carrots, onion, tomato and garlic cooking for 5 minutes or until tender, stir occasionally.
4. Add in the seasonings, couscous and cook until heated thoroughly for 2 minutes.

SMOOTHIE - Ginger Turmeric
Servings – 2   Prep – 10 mins   Cook – 0 mins

1 large banana

1 cup nut milk

1 cup pineapple, frozen or fresh

1 tbsp ginger root, grated

¼ to ½ tsp ground turmeric

1 inch aloe vera, fresh

Directions
Place all ingredients in a high speed blender.

Lunch

Grilled Chicken or Seafood
Servings – 4   Prep – 15 mins   Cook – 10 mins

4 4-6 oz grilled chicken or seafood, cooked

Greek Salad
Servings – 4   Prep – 20 mins   Cook – 0 mins

10 pitted Kalamata olives
2 tomatoes cut into wedges
1 tbsp parsley, minced
½ cup onions, sliced thinly
½ cup cucumbers, sliced thinly
½ cup green bell peppers,
  sliced thinly
½ cup red bell peppers, sliced thinly
½ cup crumbled feta cheese

Dressing:
1 small clove garlic, minced
1 tbsp fresh lemon juice
½ tsp fresh oregano, minced
¼ cup of extra virgin olive oil

Directions:
1. Spread Romaine lettuce on a platter and arrange tomato wedges.
2. Combine the onions, peppers, parsley, half of feta cheese and cucumbers in a bowl. Spread over tomato and lettuce, top with olives and remaining feta cheese.
3. Whisk the oil, lemon juice, garlic and oregano together to make the dressing. Drizzle over the salad and toss before serving.

Optional: See Condiment Section at end of chapter for Olive Oil Vinaigrette.

Dinner

Indian Chickpeas in a Bowl
Servings – 4   Prep – 15 mins   Cook – 15 mins

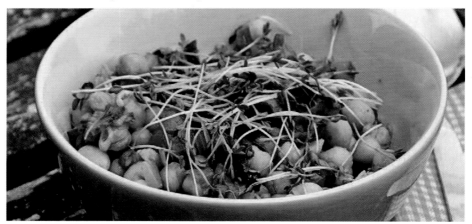

2 cans chickpeas rinsed and
  drained (or 4 cups cooked)
1 tomato, chopped
½ cup red onion, chopped
3 cloves garlic, pressed

¼ tsp chili powder
1 tsp turmeric
¼ tsp cayenne pepper (optional)
1 tbsp olive oil
½ cup watercress

Optional Serving Suggestions
1 cup cooked brown rice with avocado, sliced

Directions
1. Sauté onion 5 mins in 1 tbsp olive oil until slightly caramelized.
2. Add onion, garlic, chili powder, turmeric, cayenne pepper until fragrant.
3. Add chickpeas and tomato slowly. Reduce to medium heat for 5 mins. Stir gently. To serve, spoon generous portions in a bowl and top with watercress or optional serving suggestions.

Dessert

Chocolate Avocado Pudding with Sea Salt

Servings – 4   Prep – 10 mins   Cook – 0 mins

A decadent dessert that is rich in chocolate, creamy and healthy.
Dairy-free, vegan and paleo.

2 large avocados, chilled
½ cup full fat coconut milk
⅓ cup raw cacao powder

⅓ cup honey
2 tsp vanilla extract
Sprinkle with sea salt and/or nuts

Directions

1. Slice the avocados in half and remove the pit. Scoop out the flesh and put in a food processor.
2. Add the coconut milk, raw cacao powder, honey and vanilla extract until smooth and creamy. Scrape the sides as needed.
3. Pour chocolate avocado pudding into individual serving bowls. Sprinkle with sea salt or other topping of your choice.

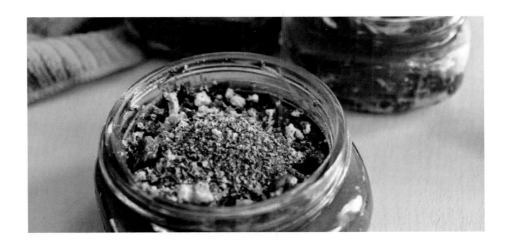

Bonus Recipes

Smoothie Options

Apple Cinnamon Smoothie
Servings – 4   Prep – 10 mins   Cook – 0 mins

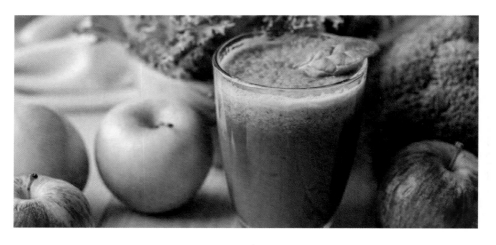

2 cups chard
2 cups almond milk
2 cups chopped apples

1 banana
¼ tsp cinnamon
½ tsp maca powder

Directions
Place all ingredients in high speed blender until liquid. Serve over ice.

Basic Green Smoothie

Servings – 4   Prep – 10 mins   Cook – 0 mins

4 cups spinach
1 cucumber
2 apples

6 leaves fresh mint
1 lemon

Directions

Place all ingredients in high speed blender until liquid. Serve over ice and drink right away.

Berry Citrus Blast with Lavender SMOOTHIE

Servings – 4   Prep – 10 mins   Cook – 0 mins

1 banana
3/4 cup frozen blueberries
1 orange, peeled
1 tbsp dried lavender
½ - ¾ cup water, as needed

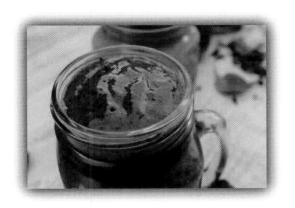

Directions

Place all ingredients in high speed blender until liquid. Serve over ice and enjoy.

Beet Limeade SMOOTHIE

Servings – 4   Prep – 10 mins   Cook – 0 mins

2 to 3 leaves chard
1 lime, juice
1 cucumber

½ red beet
1 apple

Directions

Place all ingredients in high speed blender until liquid. Serve over ice.

Acai Berry with Hemp SMOOTHIE

Servings – 4   Prep – 10 mins   Cook – 0 mins

1 cup acai berries
  Or 4 tbsp acai powder
1 cup mixed berries
1 tbsp hemp seeds

1 cup liquid (nut milk or water)
1 lemon, peeled
½ tsp maca powder
Splash vanilla extract

Directions

Place all ingredients in high speed blender. Serve over ice and drink right away.

Condiments/Dressings Options

Tomato-Cucumber Relish

Servings – 4   Prep – 20 mins   Cook – 0 mins

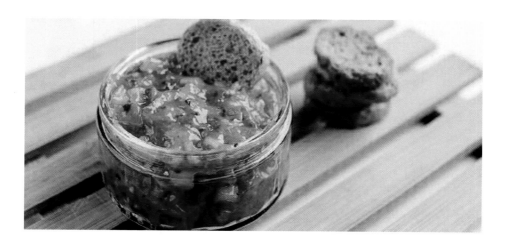

½ cup tomato, chopped
½ cup cucumber, chopped
¼ tsp dried mint

Freshly-ground black pepper and salt to taste

Directions:
1. Combine all ingredients in a blender and use low setting for 30 seconds.
2. Season with salt and pepper to taste

Olive Oil Vinaigrette
Servings –4 to 6 people   Prep – 10 mins   Cook – 0 mins

2 tbsp balsamic vinegar
2 tbsp red wine vinegar
1 tbsp fresh lemon juice
1 clove garlic, minced

1 tsp salt
½ cup of extra virgin olive oil
Dash freshly-ground black pepper

Directions
1. Combine vinegars, lemon juice, salt, garlic and pepper in a small bowl.
2. Whisk above with olive oil until well-blended. Serve with your salad of choice.

Dijon Lemon Mustard
Servings – 4   Prep – 10 mins   Cook – 0 mins

6 tbsp mustard seeds
4 tbsp lemon juice
3 tsp lemon zest
¼ cup extra virgin olive oil
¼ cup distilled white vinegar

¼ cup dry white wine (optional)
1 clove garlic, finely minced
½ tsp salt
¼ tsp black pepper
1 tbsp minced oregano

Directions

1. Blend all dry ingredients.
2. Add remaining ingredients. Blend again.
3. Cover and refrigerate for 5+ hours.
4. Can store for 3-4 weeks.

Dessert Options

Multi Seed Superfood Balls

Servings – 12   Prep – 15 mins   Cook – 0 mins

Balls:

1 cup pecans, toasted
¾ cup dates, finely chopped
¼ cup cacao
2 tbsp cacao nibs
2 tbsp flaxseeds

2 tbsp chia seeds
2 tbsp goji berries
2 tbsp cranberries
½ cup coconut flakes

Toppings: Hemp seeds, coconut flakes (toasted optional), cacao nibs

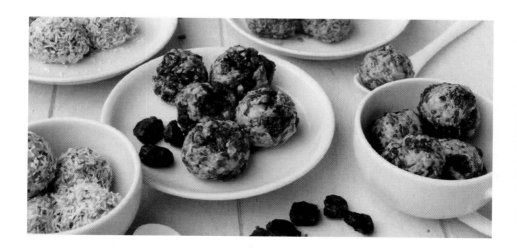

Directions
1. Place pecans in a food processor and gently process. Add remaining ball ingredients
2. Blend until mixture sticks together.
3. Roll mixture into small balls and then roll around in desired toppings.
4. Store balls in an air-tight container in the refrigerator for up to 1 week.

Trail Mix
Servings – 10   Prep – 5 mins   Cook – 0 min

½ cup dark chocolate drops
  (at least 65% cacao)
1/3 cup pistachios
1/3 cup cashew
1/3 cup walnut
1/3 cup almond
1/3 cup peanuts
1/3 cup pecans
¾ cup dried fruit, chopped
  (cherries, blueberries)

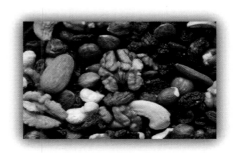

Directions:
Lightly toast nuts in the oven. Add ingredients and mix.

Chocolate Truffles with Sweet Orange
Servings – 12   Prep – 50 mins   Cook – 0 mins

Truffle filling
1 cup cocoa powder, unsweetened
1 tbsp cup coconut cream
¼ cup orange juice
1 tbsp orange zest
2 tbsp honey
Chocolate coating
1 cup cacoa powder

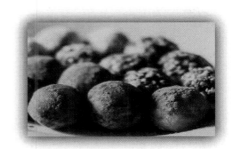

Directions

1. *Filling*: Combine ingredients in a blender, blend well.
2. When combined, place mixture in the freezer for about 45 mins. It needs to be firm enough to be scooped into balls. Adjust coconut cream as needed.
3. With a cookie or ice cream scoop, place balls on a lined baking sheet and place in the freezer for at least 30 minutes.
4. *Coating*: Roll balls in cocoa powder. Return to freezer for one hour before eating
5. Keep truffles in sealed container in freezer.

Kale, Cucumber and Apple Smoothie

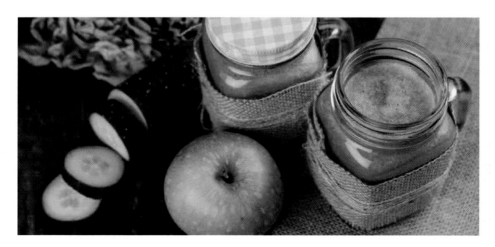

KEY 10
Nutrition is Essential in Cancer Treatment

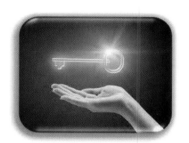

Chapter 10
Nutrition is Essential in Cancer Treatment

"Insanity is doing the same thing over and over and expecting different results."
Albert Einstein, PhD, Nobel laureate

FROM NATURE'S PHARMACY: Grapefruit

The cynical comedians comment: "grapefruit is neither grape nor fruit". Sugar loving Americans avoid grapefruit due to its tart flavor. Yet grapefruit is a warehouse of known and unknown nutritional therapeutics. Grapefruit is a rich source of vitamins A and C, pectin, potassium, and other phytochemicals. Grapefruit helps to <u>modify insulin resistance</u> and lower insulin flow, which is a major victory for cancer patients.[1] Obese research subjects who ate a half grapefruit before each meal for 12 weeks had substantially more weight loss than placebo group. Regular intake of grapefruit helps to <u>lower the risk for hypertension and heart disease</u>. [2] Grapefruit can help to prevent kidney stones, slow the aging process through its antioxidant content, and <u>even prevent cancer through the lycopene</u> content in red grapefruit. [3]

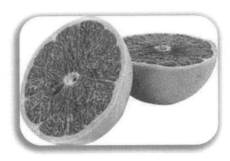

Grapefruit contains a rich assortment of flavonols, including naringin and furanocoumarins which are good for the body, but affect the way the liver breaks down prescription drugs. Grapefruit is good for human health, but <u>can affect the pharmacokinetics of how your body processes drugs</u>, hence work with your doctor and pharmacist if taking medication. [4] Grapefruit is a wonderful palate cleanser after a meal.

Adjuvant (helpful) nutrition and traditional oncology are synergistic, not antagonistic. While we have detailed the limitations of traditional oncology in Key 1, there is compelling evidence that nutrition is the missing modality in comprehensive cancer treatment. Restrained tumor killing in combination with changing the cellular environment through nutrition holds promise as 21st century cancer treatment. The advantages in using an aggressive nutrition program in comprehensive cancer treatment are, in this critical order of importance:

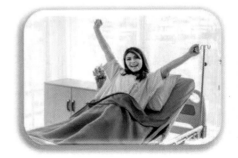

1) prevent or treat malnutrition

2) reducing the toxicity of medical therapy while making chemotherapy and radiation more selectively toxic to the tumor cells

3) stimulating immune function

4) selectively starving the tumor

5) nutrients acting as biological response modifiers to assist host defense mechanisms and improve outcome in cancer therapy.

Nutrients Alone Can Reverse Pre-Cancerous Lesions

Cancer is not an "on or off" switch. No one goes to bed on Sunday night perfectly healthy and then wakes up Monday morning with stage 4 colon cancer metastasis to the liver. Cancer takes months, and probably years to develop. Research has shown that, in the early stages of cancer cell development, nutrients alone can reverse "pre-malignant" cancers[5], which under the microscope are identical to cancer cells, yet have not invaded beyond their own "turf". As the bowling ball of cancer begins its hazardous deterioration downhill, the body has built-in mechanisms to

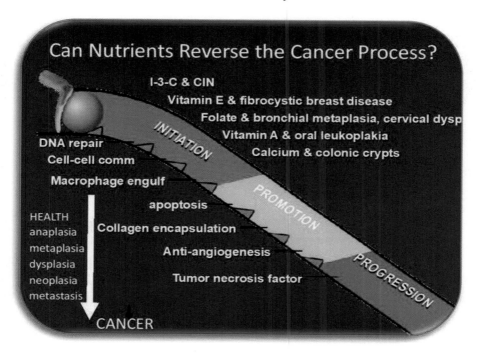

stop this process, including DNA repair, cell-to-cell communication, macrophage engulfment, tumor necrosis factor, collagen encapsulation, and anti-angiogenesis agents to shut down the making of new blood vessels from the tumor.

This concept is very pivotal to the notion that nutrition can improve outcome in cancer treatment. For decades, researchers have held the notion that "once the cell turns cancerous, only forceful eradication can help the patient." Maybe not. Pre-cancerous conditions, such as oral leukoplakia, bronchial metaplasia, and colonic crypts, can be reversed by nutrients alone. Once cancer has deteriorated to stage 4 malignancy with extensive metastasis, the patient needs appropriate medical care to selectively reduce tumor burden.

HOW CAN NUTRIENTS AFFECT THE CANCER PROCESS?

Shklar, G., Alternative & Complementary Therapies, vol.2, no.3, p.156, May 1996
-inhibit angiogenesis
-dysregulate mutant p53 oncogene
-alter immune cytokines
Schwartz, JL, Cancer Prevention Intl., vol.3, p.37, 1997
-upregulate DNA repair
-augment programmed cell death (apoptosis)
Prasad, KN, et al., Arch.Otolaryngol.Head Neck Surg., vol.119, p.1133, Oct.1993
-regulate gene expression
-induce growth inhibition in cancer
-alter cell differentiation
Lupulescu, A., Intl.J.Vit.Nutr.Res., vol.63, p.3, 1993
-A, C, E regulators of cell differentiation, membrane biogenesis, DNA synthesis
-A, C, E may be cytotoxic and cytostatic in certain cell system
-affect oncogenes
Poppel, GV, et al., Cancer Letters, vol.114, p.195, 1997
-immune stimulation
-enhancement of cell to cell communication, defuse carcinogens, etc.

Our 37 trillion cells in the human body are constantly dividing. The DNA, which contains the body's blueprints to make a completely new you, must "unzip" the spiral staircase of chromosomes, then duplicate itself exactly, then "re-zip" the spiral staircase of DNA. This process occurs billions of times daily. The chance for a mistake is quite high, which is why our bodies have many mechanisms in place to correct mistakes in the beginning. Yet, if the mistake cell continues to deteriorate through its many different shades of cancer; including anaplasia, dysplasia, and metaplasia, then the final stage of neoplasia might occur.

As this process is deteriorating, nutrients have been shown to not only arrest the slippery slide toward cancer, but also to reverse the damage and help the body to generate healthy cells from pre-malignant cancers. In high doses:

- folate and B-12 can reverse bronchial metaplasia[6] or cervical dysplasia
- beta-carotene[7] and vitamin A can reverse oral leukoplakia[8]; so can vitamin E[9]
- selenium can reverse pre-cancerous mouth lesions[10]
- vitamin C[11] and calcium can reverse colon polyps[12]
- vitamins A, C, and E reversed colorectal adenomas[13]
- vitamin E can reverse benign breast disease, such as fibrocystic breast disease, which increases the risk for breast cancer by 50-80%[14]
- vitamin E and beta-carotene injected into the tumor reversed mouth cancer in animals[15]

Pre-malignant and malignant cells look almost identical under the microscope. Since nutrients can reverse pre-malignant cells, it becomes entirely probable that nutrients can help to re-regulate malignant and metastatic cells. Maybe we don't have to kill all the cancer cells in order to cure the cancer patient. The best combination is selective tumor debulking along with re-regulation of the host defense mechanisms through the protocols described throughout this book.

Why Use Nutrition in Cancer Treatment
1) Avoiding malnutrition

40% or more of cancer patients actually die from malnutrition, not from the cancer.[16] Nutrition therapy is essential to arrest malnutrition. Among the more effective non-nutritional approaches to reverse cancer cachexia is hydrazine sulfate. Hydrazine sulfate is a relatively non-toxic drug that shuts down energy metabolism in cancer cells. Hydrazine is available through numerous vendors on the web. Protocol is to take 60 mg capsules: first 3 days 1 cap at breakfast, day 4-6 take 1 cap at breakfast and supper, day 7-45 take 3 caps TID (3x/day), off for 1 week. Contraindications are like those of an MAO inhibitor: no aged cheese, yogurt, brewer's yeast, raisins, sausage (tyramine content), excessive B-6, or overripe bananas.

Most of the scientific literature shows that weight loss drastically increases the mortality rate for most types of cancer, while also lowering the response to chemotherapy. [17] Chemo and radiation therapy are sufficient biological stressors alone to induce malnutrition.[18]

In the early years of oncology, it was thought that one could starve the tumor out of the host. Pure malnutrition (cachexia) is responsible for somewhere between 22% and 67% of all cancer deaths. Up to 80% of all cancer patients have reduced levels of serum albumin, which is a leading indicator of protein and calorie malnutrition.[19] Dietary protein restriction in the cancer patient does not affect the composition or growth rate of the

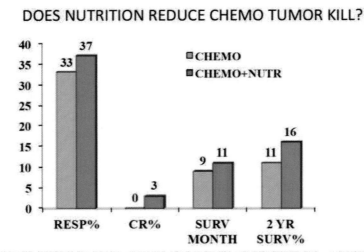

DOES NUTRITION REDUCE CHEMO TUMOR KILL?

STUDY: 136 NSCLC patients stage 3-4 randomized to chemo (paclitaxel + carbo) or chemo + nutr (6100 mg C, 1050 mg dl E, 60 mg beta carot; Kaplan-Meier surv method "These results do not support the concern that antioxidants might protect cancer cells from the free radical damage induced by chemotherapy." *J.Am.Coll.Nutr., 24, 1, 16, 2005*

tumor, but does restrict the patient's well-being.[20]

Total parenteral nutrition (TPN, feeding through a tube that is connected to the patient's blood supply) improves tolerance to chemotherapeutic agents and immune responses.[21] Malnourished cancer patients who were provided TPN had a mortality rate of 11%, while a comparable group without TPN feeding had a 100% mortality rate.[22] Pre-operative TPN in patients undergoing surgery for gastrointestinal cancer provided general reduction in the incidence of wound infection, pneumonia, major complications, and mortality.[23] Patients who were the most malnourished experienced a 33% mortality and 46% morbidity rate, while those patients who were properly nourished had a 3% mortality rate with an 8% morbidity rate.

In 20 adult hospitalized patients on TPN, the mean daily vitamin C needs were 975 mg, which is over 16 times the RDA, with the range being 350-2,250 mg.[24] Of the 139 lung cancer patients studied, most tested deficient or scorbutic (clinical vitamin C deficiency).[25] Another study of cancer patients found that 46% tested scorbutic, while 76% were below

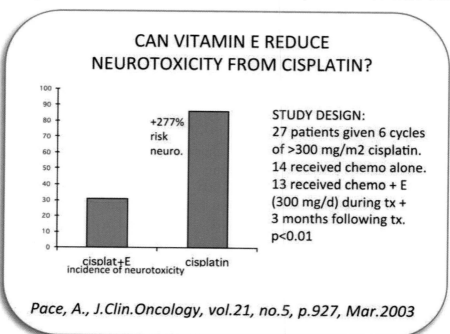

CAN VITAMIN E REDUCE NEUROTOXICITY FROM CISPLATIN?

+277% risk neuro.

STUDY DESIGN:
27 patients given 6 cycles of >300 mg/m2 cisplatin.
14 received chemo alone.
13 received chemo + E (300 mg/d) during tx + 3 months following tx.
p<0.01

cisplat+E   cisplatin
incidence of neurotoxicity

Pace, A., J.Clin.Oncology, vol.21, no.5, p.927, Mar.2003

acceptable levels for serum ascorbate.[26] Experts now recommend the value of nutritional supplements, especially in patients who require prolonged TPN support.[27]

2) Reducing the toxic effects of chemo & radiation

Properly nourished patients experience less nausea, malaise, immune suppression, hair loss, and organ toxicity than patients on routine oncology programs. Antioxidants like beta carotene, vitamin C, vitamin E, glutathione, and selenium appear to enhance the effectiveness of chemo, radiation, and hyperthermia, while minimizing damage to the patient's normal cells; thus making therapy more of a "selective toxin." An optimally-nourished cancer patient can better tolerate the rigors of cytotoxic therapy. Charles Simone, MD has published a peer reviewed meta-analysis of the world's literature on supplement use during chemo and radiation.[28] Analyzing 50 clinical trials involving 8500 cancer patients, nutrients were found to enhance outcome in cancer patients treated with chemo and radiation.

In a separate review of the world's peer reviewed scientific literature, Keith Block, MD examined 33 studies involving 2400 cancer patients and found that antioxidant supplements reduced the toxicity of the chemo allowing patients to complete their treatment cycles; and there was no reduction in tumor kill from the chemo.[29]

In many of my patients, using nutrition supplements while undergoing chemo and radiation has had a profound effect on improving patient quality of life and minimizing "collateral damage" to the patient's body. Oncologists often prescribe chemo to the "therapeutic brink of death", meaning the patient's immune system is so compromised that death by infection is very possible. By using nutrition supplements in conjunction with chemo and radiation, tumor kill is unaffected while the patient's immune system remains intact.

3) Bolster immune functions

When the doctor says "We think we got it all", what he or she is really saying is "We have destroyed all DETECTABLE cancer cells, and now it is up to your immune system to find and destroy the cancer cells that inevitably remain in your body." A billion cancer cells are about the size of the page number at the top of this page. We must rely on the capabilities of the 20 trillion cells that compose an intact immune system to destroy the undetectable cancer cells that remain after medical therapy. There is an abundance of data linking nutrient intake to the quality and quantity of immune factors that fight cancer.[30]

4) Sugar feeds cancer

Tumors are primarily obligate glucose metabolizers, meaning "sugar feeders".[31] Americans not only consume about 20% of their calories from refined sugars (sucrose, fructose, high fructose corn syrup), but often manifest poor glucose tolerance curves due to stress, eating too often, obesity, low chromium and fiber intake, and sedentary lifestyles.

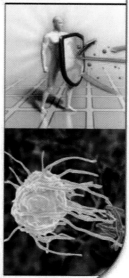

IMMUNOLOGY 101A

function: recognize self from non-self
major histocompatibility complex (MHC) or
human leukocyte antigen (HLA in humans)
IMMUNE SURVEILLANCE IS CRITICAL

destruction via: phagocytosis
oxidative burst, membrane pen
enzymatic breakdown

Mucosal/mechanical (skin, membranes,tears)
Lymphatic: nodes, spleen,Peyer's patches (GI)
Non-Specific: phagocytosis,reticulo-endothelial,complement
Specific: produced in bone marrow
    Cell Mediated: T-lymphocytes (killer,helper,suppressor)
    Humoral: B-lymphocytes mature to antibodies
    (immunoglobulin GAMED); react to antigens+complement
    Natural Killer cells: from bone marrow
Cytokines (proteins) for communication
    TNF, interferon,interleukin 1-6, colony stim.factor
40-50% of immune system surrounds GI tract
Bock, ROAD TO IMMUNITY, Pocket, NY 1997
Myrvik, MODERN NUTRITION,Lea,Phila, 1994

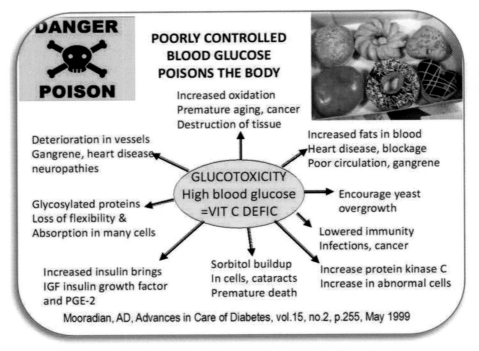

DANGER

POISON

POORLY CONTROLLED BLOOD GLUCOSE POISONS THE BODY

Increased oxidation
Premature aging, cancer
Destruction of tissue

Deterioration in vessels
Gangrene, heart disease
neuropathies

Increased fats in blood
Heart disease, blockage
Poor circulation, gangrene

GLUCOTOXICITY
High blood glucose
=VIT C DEFIC

Glycosylated proteins
Loss of flexibility &
Absorption in many cells

Encourage yeast
overgrowth

Lowered immunity
Infections, cancer

Increased insulin brings
IGF insulin growth factor
and PGE-2

Sorbitol buildup
In cells, cataracts
Premature death

Increase protein kinase C
Increase in abnormal cells

Mooradian, AD, Advances in Care of Diabetes, vol.15, no.2, p.255, May 1999

5) Nutrients as biological response modifiers (BRM)

In December of 1971 Richard Nixon launched the "war on cancer" with a promise of a cure for a major cancer by the Bicentennial of 1976. Researchers began an earnest quest for a "magic bullet" or <u>biological response modifier</u> to cure cancer. We still don't have a cure for any major cancer, but we do know a lot more about cancer and how the body can defend itself. Nature provides us with a host of BRMs to prevent and reverse cancer. It is about time that we started harnessing these incredible agents.

Certain nutrients, like selenium, vitamin K, vitamin E succinate, and the fatty acid EPA, appear to have the ability to slow down the unregulated growth of cancer. Various nutrition factors, including vitamin A, D, folacin, bioflavonoids, and soybeans, have been shown to alter the genetic expression of tumors.

Putting It All Together

Finnish oncologists used high doses of nutrients along with chemo and radiation for lung cancer patients. Normally, lung cancer is a "poor prognostic" malignancy, with a 1% expected survival at 30 months under normal treatment. In this study, however, 8 of the 18 patients (44%) that were given nutrition supplements were still alive 6 years after therapy.[32]

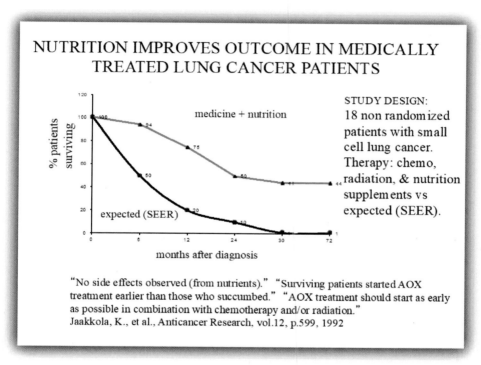

NUTRITION IMPROVES OUTCOME IN MEDICALLY
TREATED LUNG CANCER PATIENTS

STUDY DESIGN:
18 non randomized patients with small cell lung cancer. Therapy: chemo, radiation, & nutrition supplements vs expected (SEER).

"No side effects observed (from nutrients)." "Surviving patients started AOX treatment earlier than those who succumbed." "AOX treatment should start as early as possible in combination with chemotherapy and/or radiation."
Jaakkola, K., et al., Anticancer Research, vol.12, p.599, 1992

In a non-randomized clinical trial, Drs. Hoffer and Pauling instructed patients to follow a reasonable cancer diet (unprocessed foods low in fat, dairy, and sugar), coupled with therapeutic doses of vitamins and minerals.[33] All 129 patients in this study received concomitant oncology care. The control group of 31 patients who did not receive nutrition support lived an average of less than 6 months. The group of 98 cancer patients who did receive the diet and supplement program were categorized into 3 groups:

- Poor responders (n=19) or 20% of treated group. Average lifespan of 10 months, or a 75% improvement over the control group.
- Good responders (n=47), who had various cancers, including leukemia, lung, liver, and pancreas; had an average lifespan of 72 months (6 years) or a 1,200% improvement in lifespan.
- Good female responders (n=32), with involvement of reproductive areas (breast, cervix, ovary, uterus); had an average lifespan of over 10 years, or a 2,100% improvement in lifespan. Many were still alive at the end of the study.

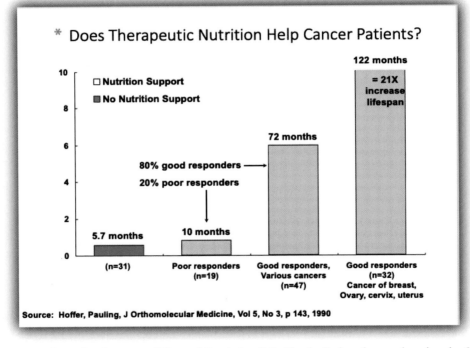

Source: Hoffer, Pauling, J Orthomolecular Medicine, Vol 5, No 3, p 143, 1990

Oncologists at West Virginia Medical School randomized 65 patients with transitional cell carcinoma of the bladder into either the "one-per-day" vitamin supplement providing the RDA, or into a group which received the RDA supplement plus 40,000 iu of vitamin A, 100 mg of B-6, 2,000 mg of vitamin C, 400 iu of vitamin E, and 90 mg of zinc. At 10 months, tumor recurrence was 80% in the control group (RDA supplement) and 40% in the experimental "megavitamin" group. Five year projected tumor recurrence was 91% for controls and 41% for "megavitamin" patients. Essentially, high dose nutrients cut tumor recurrence in half.[34]

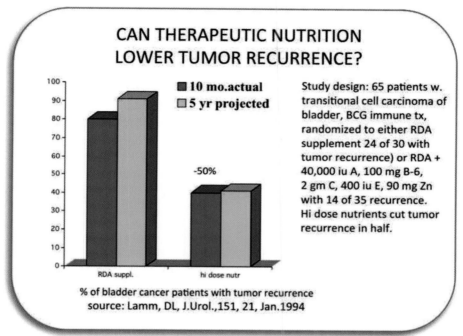

CAN THERAPEUTIC NUTRITION LOWER TUMOR RECURRENCE?

■ 10 mo.actual
□ 5 yr projected

-50%

RDA suppl.   hi dose nutr

% of bladder cancer patients with tumor recurrence
source: Lamm, DL, J.Urol.,151, 21, Jan.1994

Study design: 65 patients w. transitional cell carcinoma of bladder, BCG immune tx, randomized to either RDA supplement 24 of 30 with tumor recurrence) or RDA + 40,000 iu A, 100 mg B-6, 2 gm C, 400 iu E, 90 mg Zn with 14 of 35 recurrence. Hi dose nutrients cut tumor recurrence in half.

Of the 200 cancer patients studied who experienced "spontaneous regression", 87% made a major change in diet, mostly vegetarian in nature, 55% used some form of detoxification, and 65% used nutritional supplements.[35]

Researchers at Tulane University compared survival in patients who used the macrobiotic diet versus patients who continued with their standard Western lifestyle. Of 1,467 pancreatic cancer patients who made no changes in diet, 146 (1%) were alive after one year, while 12 of the 23 matched pancreatic cancer patients (52%) consuming macrobiotic foods were still alive after one year.[36] In examining the diet and lifespan of 675 lung cancer patients over the course of 6 years, researchers found that the more vegetables consumed, the longer the lung cancer patient lived.[37] By adding an aggressive nutrition component to your comprehensive cancer treatment program, you improve the odds for a complete remission/regression and probably add significantly to the quality and quantity of life.

Keith Block, MD has published a 12 year study showing a doubling of lifespan in 90 metastatic breast cancer patients employing nutrition as an essential component in comprehensive cancer treatment.[38]

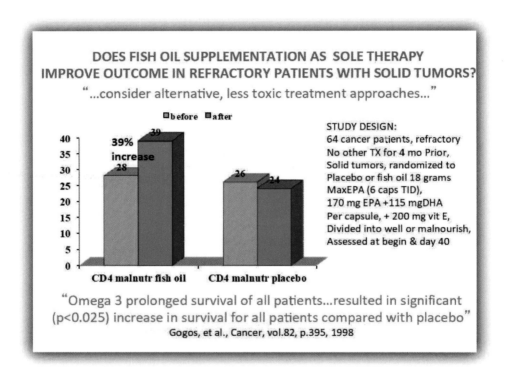

DOES FISH OIL SUPPLEMENTATION AS SOLE THERAPY IMPROVE OUTCOME IN REFRACTORY PATIENTS WITH SOLID TUMORS?

"...consider alternative, less toxic treatment approaches..."

before after

39% increase

STUDY DESIGN:
64 cancer patients, refractory
No other TX for 4 mo Prior,
Solid tumors, randomized to
Placebo or fish oil 18 grams
MaxEPA (6 caps TID),
170 mg EPA +115 mgDHA
Per capsule, + 200 mg vit E,
Divided into well or malnourish,
Assessed at begin & day 40

CD4 malnutr fish oil   CD4 malnutr placebo

"Omega 3 prolonged survival of all patients...resulted in significant ($p<0.025$) increase in survival for all patients compared with placebo"
Gogos, et al., Cancer, vol.82, p.395, 1998

Nutritional Oncology Program Should Include:

1) Food. If the gut works and if the patient can consume enough food through the mouth, then this is the primary route for nourishing the patient. The diet for the cancer patient should be high in plant food (grains, legumes, nuts, seeds, seaweed, mushrooms, colorful vegetables, fruit, medicinal spices), unprocessed (shop the perimeter of the grocery store), low in salt, fat, and sugar, with adequate protein (1 gram/kilogram body weight).

2) Supplements. Additional vitamins, minerals, amino acids, food extracts (i.e. bovine cartilage), conditionally essential nutrients (i.e. fish, flax, and borage oil; coenzyme Q-10), and botanicals (i.e. echinacea, goldenseal, astragalus) can enhance the patient's recuperative powers.

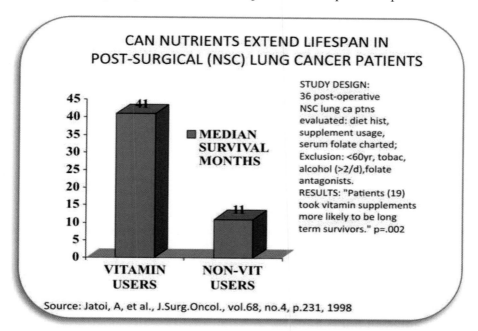

CAN NUTRIENTS EXTEND LIFESPAN IN POST-SURGICAL (NSC) LUNG CANCER PATIENTS

MEDIAN SURVIVAL MONTHS

STUDY DESIGN: 36 post-operative NSC lung ca ptns evaluated: diet hist, supplement usage, serum folate charted; Exclusion: <60yr, tobac, alcohol (>2/d),folate antagonists. RESULTS: "Patients (19) took vitamin supplements more likely to be long term survivors." p=.002

Source: Jatoi, A, et al., J.Surg.Oncol., vol.68, no.4, p.231, 1998

3) Total parenteral nutrition (TPN). There are many cancer patients who are so malnourished (weight loss of 10% below usual body weight within a 1-month period and/or serum albumin below 2.5 mg/dl) that we must interrupt this deterioration with TPN. When the patient cannot or will not eat adequately, TPN can be an invaluable life raft during crucial phases of cancer treatment.

4) Assessment. Means of assessment include: health history form to detect lifestyle risk factors; physician's examination; anthropometric measurements of height, weight, and percent body fat; calorimeter measurement of basal metabolic needs; and various other laboratory tests.

5) Education. A pro-active patient can help reverse the underlying causative factors of cancer.

6) Research. Those who advance the knowledge base have a responsibility to properly gather data and report their findings to the world.

Summary

America has spent over $200 billion in research and $4 trillion in therapies over the past 48-year war on cancer with few minor victories to claim. Adding nutrition and other modalities mentioned in this book can dramatically improve the quality and quantity of life with improved chances for a complete remission. 42% of Americans living today will get cancer in their lifetime. By adding nutrition therapies to modern oncology, we can improve the outlook for those millions of cancer patients.

For more information about why nutrition is essential in cancer treatment go to GettingHealthier.com.

PATIENT PROFILE

J.H. was a wasting 38-year old male with advanced lymphoma when he was admitted to our hospital as a medical emergency, having failed prior therapies. He was dying more from malnutrition than the cancer. We put him on total parenteral nutrition, with a disease-specific formula that is higher in protein and fats and lower in glucose than standard TPN formulas. Within a month, he was able to eat solid foods. He rebounded from his malnutrition so that he could resume chemo. Within 6 months he was disease-free. Eight years later, still in remission, he attended our Celebrate Life festival and planted a tree.

ENDNOTES

[1] https://www.ncbi.nlm.nih.gov/pubmed/16579728
[2] https://www.ncbi.nlm.nih.gov/pubmed/22304836
[3] https://www.ncbi.nlm.nih.gov/pubmed/20394143

[4] https://www.sciencedirect.com/topics/pharmacology-toxicology-and-pharmaceutical-science/grapefruit

[5] . Singh, VN, Am.J.Clin.Nutr., vol.53, p.386S, 1991

[6] . Heimburger, DC, JAMA, vol.259, no.10, p.1525, Mar.11, 1988

[7] . Toma, S., Oncology, vol.49, p.77, 1992

[8] . Stich, HF, Am.J.Clin.Nutr., vol.53, p.298S, 1991

[9] . Benner, SE, J.National Cancer Institute, vol.85, no.1, p.44, Jan.1993

[10] . Toma, S., Cancer Detection & Prevention, vol.15, no.6, p.491, 1991

[11] DeCosse, JJ, Surgery, vol.78, no.5, p.608, Nov.1975

[12] . Wargovich, MJ, et al., Gastroenterology, vol.103, p.92, 1992; see also Steinbach, G., Gastroenterology, vol.106, p.1162, 1994

[13] . Paganelli, GM, J. National Cancer Institute, vol.84,no.1, p.47, Jan.1992

[14] . Krieger, N, American J. Epidemiology, vol.135, no.6, p.619, 1992; see also London, SJ, JAMA, vol.267, no.7, p.941, Feb.1992

[15] . Shklar, G., Nutr Cancer, vol.12, p.321, 1989

[16]. Grant, JP, Nutrition, 6, 4, 6S, July 1990 suppl

[17]. Dewys, WD, et al., Cachexia and cancer treatment, Amer J Med, 69, 491-5, Oct.1980

[18]. Wilmore, DW, Catabolic illness, strategies for recovery, N Engl J Med, 1991, 325:10:695-702

[19]. Dreizen, S., et al., Malnutrition in cancer, Postgrad Med, 87, 1, 163-7, Jan.1990

[20]. Lowry, SF, et al., Nutrient restriction in cancer patients, Surg Forum, 28, 143-9, 1977

[21]. Eys, JV, Total parenteral nutrition and response to cytotoxic therapies, Cancer, 43, 2030-7, 1979

[22]. Harvey, KB, et al., Morbidity in parenterally-nourished cancer patients, Cancer, 43, 2065-9, 1979

[23]. Muller, JM, et al., Nutritional status as a factor in GI cancer morbidity, Lancet, 68-73, Jan.9, 1982

[24]. Abrahamian, V., et al., Ascorbic acid requirements in hospital patients, JPEN, 7, 5, 465-8, 1983

[25]. Anthony, HM, et al., Vitamin C status of lung cancer patients, Brit J Ca, 46, 354-9, 1982

[26]. Cheraskin, E., Scurvy in cancer patients?, J Altern Med, 18-23, Feb.1986

[27]. Hoffman, FA, Micronutrient status of cancer patients, Cancer, 55, 1 sup.1, 295-9, Jan.1, 1985

[28] . https://www.ncbi.nlm.nih.gov/pubmed/17405678

[29] https://www.ncbi.nlm.nih.gov/pubmed/18623084

[30]. Bendich, A, Chandra, RK (eds), Micronutrients and Immune Function, New York Academy of Sciences, 1990, p.587

[31]. Rothkopf, M, Fuel utilization in neoplastic disease: implications for the use of nutritional support in cancer patients, Nutrition, supp, 6:4:14-16S, 1990

[32]. Jaakkola, K., et al., Treatment with antioxidant and other nutrients in combination with chemotherapy and irradiation in patients with lung cancer, Anticancer Res 12,599-606, 1992

[33]. Hoffer, A, Pauling, L, J Orthomolecular Med, 5:3:143-154, 1990

[34]. Lamm, DL, et al., Megadose vitamin in bladder cancer, J Urol, 151:21-26, 1994

[35]. Foster, HD, Lifestyle influences on cancer regression, Int J Biosoc Res, 10:1:17-20, 1988

[36]. Carter, JP, Macrobiotic diet and cancer survival, J Amer Coll Nutr, 12:3:209-215, 1993

[37]. Goodman, MT, Vegetable consumption in lung cancer longevity, Eur J Ca, 28:2: 495-499, 1992

[38]. https://www.ncbi.nlm.nih.gov/pubmed/19470134

KEY 11
Change the Underlying Causes of the Disease

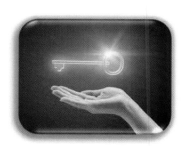

Chapter 11
Change the Underlying
Causes of the Disease

"The doctor of the future will give no medicine, but will involve the patient in the proper use of food, fresh air and exercise."
Thomas Edison, inventor with over 1000 patents

FROM NATURE'S PHARMACY: Lemons

The lemon tree is a small evergreen tree native to north India, making its appearance in Europe around 200 AD. Lemon trees grow best in a Mediterranean climate, meaning they need a hot dry summer and no frost winter. Lemons are high in vitamin C, pectin, and citric acid, which gives the lemon its characteristic flavor that makes some mouths pucker.

The unique flavor and acid in lemons have made lemons, lemon zest (the peeling), and lemon juice a favorite in foods, desserts, and drinks. Regular consumption of lemons may lower the risk for hypertension, heart disease, and favor an ideal body weight.

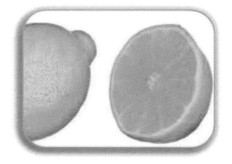

But the real magic in lemons is more subtle and lies in lemons ability to prevent kidney stones by making the urine less acidic.[1] Lemon juice is similar in pH to stomach acid, around 2, thus making lemon juice an excellent way to improve digestion. Citrus fruit in general protects against some cancers.[2] D-limonene is a compound found in lemon oil that seems to reverse cancers in animals.[3] The peel and pulp of citrus has been modified to create modified citrus pectin, which has demonstrated a broad ability to prevent and reverse various cancers in animals and humans.[4] Be careful not to chew lemons or the acid will erode the tooth enamel. Add 1-2 tablespoons of fresh squeezed lemon juice to a glass of tea or water with each meal to enhance digestion.

No one with a headache is suffering from a deficiency of aspirin. No one with cancer has a deficiency of chemo. The only way to get long term remission from any condition is to change the underlying causes of the disease.

Determining the origin of cancer could be simple or very complex. This chapter is meant to inspire you, the patient, to work with a qualified doctor to get at the root of your health problem. Cancer is a consequence of poor health. Restoring your health requires a bright and dedicated doctor to do some serious detective work.

The typical allopathic physician works within the paradigm of their training, usually meaning 7 minutes with the patient, then prescribe some medication. Doctors who solve the riddle of your health challenge are sometimes called "holistic, functional, integrative, alternative, complementary, naturopathic, etc." Call it what you will. Changing the underlying cause of your health problem is crucial.

Dale Bredesen, MD has written a brilliant book <u>THE END OF ALZHEIMER'S</u>, in which he documents the extensive work required to determine the broken systems in the body of the Alzheimer's patient and how to fix them. Point is, this is difficult but mandatory work in order to heal. This brief chapter is meant to inspire you to work with a talented doctor to restore your body's host defense mechanisms. Because "a healthy human body is self-regulating and self-repairing."

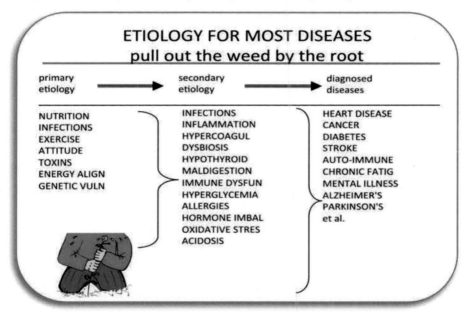

Realize the complexities of the human body. Many things can go wrong. Listed below are some of the more common health problems that eventually lead to cancer. Work with your doctor on this subject.

Get Help: Functional Medicine Practitioners

Determining the underlying causes of a disease can require brilliant detective work on the part of the doctor. Changing the underlying causes is essential, though not necessarily easy.

- The <u>Institute for Functional Medicine</u> has a website that helps you to locate a health care professional who can help you solve the mystery of etiology of disease.[5]
- The <u>American Association of Naturopathic Physicians</u> also has a website to help you find a local talented doctor.[6]
- <u>Life Extension Foundation</u> also has a listing of innovative practitioners.[7]

Oxygen: Enemy of Cancer

Humans can survive months without food, days without water, but only a few minutes without oxygen. We are aerobic creatures, requiring oxygen. For decades, heart surgeons have worked feverishly to provide adequate oxygen to surgery patients to avoid the common <u>brain damage from open heart surgery</u>.[8]

Otto Warburg, MD was a German scientist awarded the Nobel prize in 1931 for his discovery that cancer is an anaerobic organism: "the prime cause of cancer is the replacement of the respiration of oxygen in normal body cells by a fermentation of sugar." The Warburg principle is at the foundation of the multi-million dollar PET scan device. In PET scans, the doctor injects radioactively labeled sugar into the patient's veins, then tracks the destination of that sugar, because cancer is an anaerobic sugar feeder (obligate glucose metabolizer).

The amount of oxygen that can be dissolved in human tissue is very dependent on pH, or acid/base balance. The first "domino" in poor health often involves metabolic acidosis from poor diet, toxins, stress, etc. Some researchers assess that the <u>tumor generates the acidosis</u>.[9] Other experts report that a <u>poor diet (high meat and salt) generates metabolic acidosis</u> which is the first domino to fall in the sequence of cancer.[10]

Some doctors have <u>used sodium bicarbonate</u> (baking soda) given orally to mitigate the acidosis found in many cancer patients.[11] Once the cells become slightly more acidic, less oxygen can dissolve in the tissue. Once that happens, opportunistic pathogens arise from their dormancy and begin to colonize the body, eventually resulting in some serious diseases, like cancer. Restoring the original healthy pH along with maximum oxygen saturation of tissue is crucial for long term cancer outcome.

Forest Devastation

When Europeans landed in North America around 1500, a squirrel could jump from tree to tree from the Mississippi River to the Atlantic Ocean and never touch the ground. Such were our forests. We have replaced forests with farmland and cities. In the past 8000 years humans have cut down half of the forests on earth, most of that in the 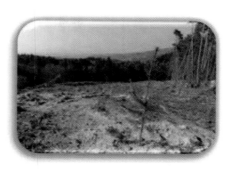 past 30 years. Trees provide humans with shade, wood, fruit, roots that prevent soil erosion, and habitat for millions of plants, animals and insects. Trees also give us oxygen. Tiny plants in the ocean (phytoplankton) generate about half the oxygen on earth, while green plants, especially trees generate the other half of our oxygen supply. The air we breathe is about 20% oxygen today, unless you live in a large polluted city, in which case you are breathing 15% oxygen. Oxygen content of the earth in prehistoric times was 30%.

Essentially, cancer seems to be some mutation that occurs when the cell can no longer breathe. Rather than suffocate, the cell switches to fermenting anaerobic "flex fuel" and continues living, at great expense to the host. There are many theories about why this shift from oxygen to low oxygen occurs: changes in cell membrane dynamics, cell to cell communication, long term nutrient deficiencies, toxic DNA hits, acidic pH, voltage drop, and more. But it is clear that making the cell more aerobic improves outcome in both traditional cancer treatment and comprehensive care that takes a whole-body approach to therapy.

Cancer can be more resistant to radiation therapy when the tumor becomes highly anaerobic (lacking oxygen). In animal studies, vitamin B3, niacin, nicotinamide was able to dramatically enhance tumor radiosensitivity, thus killing more cancer cells simply by introducing aerobic nutrients to the tissue. Hyperbaric oxygen therapy (HBOT) uses a chamber to force more oxygen into the patient's tissues. There is some evidence that HBOT is effective [12] at slowing cancer growth.

What to Do?

The ancient mystics recognized the importance of proper breathing. Meditation begins with controlling the breath. <u>Controlling breathing</u> [13] can eliminate mild to moderate anxiety. <u>Diaphragmatic breathing</u> [14] (deep belly breathing) has been shown to help control blood pressure, PTSD, IBS, insomnia, depression and more.

Proper breathing brings about a balanced ratio of oxygen and carbon dioxide, which is essential for regulating many processes in the body. Exhale all of the air in your lungs. Slowly breathe in by raising your stomach outward, then continue the inhalation process until your lungs are full...all this to a count of four. <u>Hold your breath for a count of 7,</u> [15] then exhale for a count of 8. This breathing helps to calm a person.

Normal healthy breathing should slow your breath rate to 6 breaths per minute. Not, of course, when you are exercising. This slower rate of breathing optimizes the sympathetic and parasympathetic nervous systems with an ideal blend of oxygen and carbon dioxide in the blood.

Use hyper-oxygenation. Lay down, if possible. Use deep belly breathing rapidly to the count of "one thousand and one"...count up to 30 breaths with one per second. Now stop the hyper-oxygenation process and just relax and feel the wave of serenity settle in. You have made a decent effort at bringing more oxygen to your body cells. Use this technique to relax on an airplane ride or to get to sleep at night.

EWOT. Exercise with oxygen therapy is a method of using an oxygen generator while exercising, using a stationary bike or rowing machine. <u>EWOT improves circulation</u> and reduces inflammation in chronically oxygen-starved capillaries. Good for general health and longevity. Therapeutic for cancer patients.

HBOT. Find a clinic that will help you with hyperbaric oxygen therapy, which is beneficial for everyone, particularly cancer patients, infections, wound healing, nerve damage and more.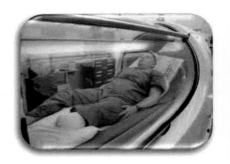

NUTRITION. Acid/base balance is a major vector driving the ability to absorb and retain oxygen in the cells. Nutrition is a major vector influencing pH. Red blood cells bring oxygen from the lungs to the cells. Nutrients required to build red blood cells include iron, copper, folate, B-12, B-6, protein, and more. Nutrients are required for the cell to use oxygen in burning food for energy; including niacin, riboflavin, thiamin, biotin, lipoic acid, CoQ. Nutrients are required to keep the cell membrane fluid and able to absorb nutrients including oxygen. Cell membranes require cholesterol, essential fats (omega 6 and 3), and avoidance of trans fats which gum up the cell membrane. Nutrients are required to release the energy from ATP in aerobic metabolism, including magnesium. What is the most important part of your car? Answer: all of it. What is the most important nutrient in the diet? Answer: all of it. More on nutrition throughout this book.

PLANT A TREE. If we continue to pollute the oceans, where phytoplankton generate half of our oxygen, then cut down the forests, which contribute the other half of our oxygen, then we are, essentially, strangling ourselves to death. The cancer epidemic of the 21st century may be somewhat related to our poor stewardship of our planet and our bodies. Good planets are hard to come by. Let's heal the planet that we steward and heal our bodies at the same time. Our cancer epidemic will subside in the process.

Infections

There are thousands of species of parasites, viruses, bacteria, fungi and more that can infect the human body. These chronic infections can lower the body's ability to heal itself. Many infections are opportunistic, meaning they take the opportunity when the body's defenses are compromised to infect the host (you).

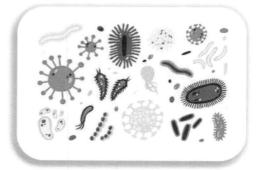

Infections can come from outside of us or inside of us, such as the gut or the mouth. Dental infections are a common cause of mysterious ailments. There are 15 million root canal procedures done annually in the US. George Meinig, DDS was one of the developers of the root canal procedure, then spent the last part of his career trying to inform professionals and the public of the <u>hazards of root canals</u>.

There are many very bright professionals who feel that cancer is merely an <u>advanced fungal infection</u> that has mutated and merged with the human DNA. Detecting the original source of the fungal infection becomes crucial.

Inflammation

Inflammation, or swelling of tissue, is at the root of many ailments. There are thousands of legitimate peer reviewed scientific studies showing the link between chronic inflammation and cancer. There are several good books by experts:

<u>INFLAMMATION NATION</u> by Sunil Pai, MD
<u>INFLAMMATION NATION</u> by Floyd Chilton, PhD

While there are many moving parts to this discussion, there are a few factors that are

Pro-inflammatory: meat, dairy, sugar, alcohol, trans fats, drugs, stress, toxins, burns, friction, elevated blood glucose and more.

Anti-inflammatory factors include fruits and vegetables, antioxidants, stress reduction, controlling insulin and blood glucose, proper fats (EPA and GLA), and many spices like turmeric and ginger.

Hypercoagulability

Blood that is thick or sticky is more likely to induce cancer. Blood should run like red wine with a very low viscosity (friction) as opposed to most Americans have blood that runs like catsup, with a high viscosity. Surgeons who get used to operating on the typical American who has thick blood and clots quickly will call a healthy person a "bleeder" because their blood is lower in viscosity…which is good for the patient's health, but tough for the surgeon to keep bleeding under control.

Techniques for lowering blood viscosity include: lower fasting blood glucose, capsaicin (hot peppers), ginger, fish oil, GLA, turmeric, and more.

Dysbiosis

The human gut contains 100 trillion microorganisms that provide us with many benefits in exchange for us providing them with "room and board". Unless things get out of whack. See the chapter on the Microbiome for more details.

Hypothyroidism

The thyroid gland is a butterfly shaped organ at the base of the neck that releases the hormones thyroxin T3 and T4, which regulate metabolism, or the burning of fuel in every cell in the body. Meaning, thyroxin affects everything. Low thyroid output, or hypothyroidism can cause fatigue, depression, constipation, sensitivity to cold, joint and muscle pain, heavy periods...and even cancer. Some experts estimate that 90% of Americans are hypothyroid. Iodine is an essential mineral in thyroid metabolism. The thyroid gland can be compromised by fluoride (in nearly all drinking water and toothpaste), chlorine (water supply), plastics in our drinking water (bottled water).

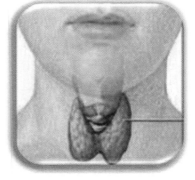

Iodine is a very unusual mineral, because it is essential in human metabolism and a selective toxin for most microbes. Early explorers would bring an iodine tablet to add to a helmet full of river water teeming with parasites and microbes. Iodine is a crucial part of the body electric, our immunity, our resistance to cancer and more.

Globally, 2 billion people suffer from iodine deficiency, which is generally obtained from seafood and seaweed.[16] Children without adequate thyroid may suffer permanent mental retardation. Hypothyroid adults develop brain fog, lowered immunity, constipation, coldness, easy weight gain. Hypothyroidism is a risk factor for post-menopausal women developing breast cancer.[17]

Maldigestion

The human digestive tract is a marvel to behold. Somehow we take a carrot or a steak and render bulk food into something that can be absorbed into the bloodstream to feed our cells. Miraculous by anyone's standards. And fraught with breakdown when consuming the Standard American Diet (SAD). We need teeth to chew the food. Americans over age 50 have lost an average of 8 teeth. Many people suffer GERD (gastro esophageal reflux disorder) with acid reflux from the stomach into the esophagus.

The stomach must start with arterial pH blood of 7.42 and churn that down to stomach acid of 2.0 pH, which is a one billion fold drop in pH. Many people do not make enough hydrochloric acid in the stomach

or amylase (starches), protease (protein), lipase (fat) in the intestines to properly digest food. Many people have damaged the lining of the small intestines creating a leaky gut, causing proteins from food to leak into the blood stream.

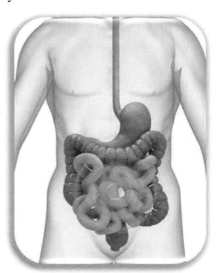

Then there is the large intestines and the 100 trillion microbes who have an important job in our digestion, vitamin production, immune system, and cross talk that regulates many functions in the human body. Any or all of this process can malfunction. Enter the need for a bright doc to fix the problem.

Immune Dysfunction

Your 20 trillion immune cells are your defense against the hostile outside world. These cells have the job of recognizing "self" from "non-self". If the immune system has been compromised, then infections, cancer and premature aging will ensue. Much of this book has the ultimate goal of restoring your immune system to full competence.

Hyperglycemia

As you have seen throughout this book, cancer is a sugar feeder, or obligate glucose metabolizer. Some therapists have taken this sound bite and banned carbohydrate foods for inducing cancer. Not so quick. The inconvenient truth is that our body can make glucose (sugar) from proteins, stored carbs (glycogen), or even fat. The real quest here is to <u>lower insulin output</u>.[18]

What is happening in most people in developed nations is insulin resistance from eating too much, too often, and the wrong food. That constant pounding of glucose and insulin on the cell membranes yields insulin resistance, which then makes the cells inside starving while there is a glut of sugar outside the cell. The ultimate therapy to fix this problem is...drum roll...stop eating. Just for a while. Intermittent fasting is the key here.

Read the chapter on Intermittent Fasting. A ketogenic diet or even fasting seems beneficial for some cancer patients, especially brain cancer. Meanwhile all cancer patients can benefit from medically supervised intermittent fasting. Narrow your eating "window". Eat your first meal at noon and last meal at 6 pm, effectively fasting for 18 hours every day. Then take one day a week and consume nothing but non-caloric fluids: water, tea, coffee. Buy a blood glucose monitoring kit at your local pharmacy. Track your blood glucose levels before and after meals and at the end of a 24 hour fast.

Additionally, there are nutrients that are required to assist insulin in getting blood glucose into the cell. Most Americans are deficient in the trace mineral chromium, which becomes part of Glucose Tolerance Factor (GTF) which works hand in hand with insulin to get glucose into the cell. Chromium supplements can have a <u>major impact on lowering blood glucose</u> for diabetics and others.[19] Vanadium is another trace mineral commonly deficient in the American diet that plays a <u>major role in blood glucose regulation</u>.[20]

Allergies

There are many adverse reactions to food and our environment. Some reactions can be swift and life threatening, such as people who are allergic to bee stings or antibiotics. Some reactions are more subtle and delayed. It helps to work with a doctor knowledgeable in this area. "One man's meat is another man's poison." Not everyone can eat every food, especially if the gut and immune system are compromised. Allergies can cause a leaky gut, or vice versa, which creates stress and infinite "decoys" of food particles in the blood that distract the immune system.

Oxidative Stress

Oxygen is essential to human life. Oxygen is also the cause of our demise. We need a healthy balance of oxygen, prooxidants (the immune system uses prooxidants to kill invaders), and antioxidants. Oxidative stress is at the root of many cancers. Oxidation can be caused by wrong foods (overcooked foods), not enough of the right foods (colorful fruits and vegetables), stress, toxins, and more.

Hormone Imbalance

The human endocrine system secretes and circulates over 50 hormones. There are male and female hormones. There are stress hormones. There are blood glucose regulating hormones. And more. As we age, many people have a decline in hormone output, especially if we are exposed to poor diet, stress, toxins, etc. Balancing hormones can be a complex but essential task in cancer recovery.

Prostate cancer patients are often put on androgen blocker drugs, as if androgen is the cause of prostate cancer. If that is the case, then every stud on Sunday TV sports would have prostate cancer because these young male athletes have a lot more androgen than the average prostate cancer patient. The problem comes when __androgen is converted__ to estrogen via the aromatase pathway. [21] Estrogen and the aromatase pathway is the problem, not androgen. These androgen blockers always lose their effectiveness against prostate cancer as the cancer becomes "__hormone independent__."[22]

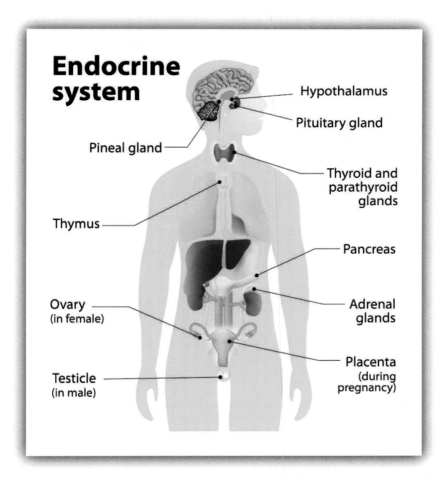

Same thing with breast cancer. Tampering with <u>estradiol and progesterone levels in a woman's body</u>, especially with synthetic hormones that do not have the same activity as bio-identical hormones, can be fraught with peril.[23] Work with your doctor on hormone balancing.

Acidosis

One of the more crucial aspects of human health is pH, or potential hydrogens. This scale shows the balance between acid and base. The pH scale exists on a logarithmic scale, meaning going from 6 to 7 is not a 16% increase, but a 10 fold or 1000% increase. Slight changes in pH dramatically affect the health of the cell and even the amount of oxygen available. Normal arterial pH in humans ranges from 7.35-7.45. Stomach acid should be 2.0 pH, while urine may be 6.0.

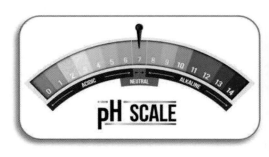

Some very bright researchers speculate that shifting the pH from an ideal of 7.42 in the arteries to a tolerable but disease inducing 7.3 may be the beginning insult that leads to lower amounts of oxygen concentrations in the tissue, which causes cells to become undifferentiated, or mutate to become anaerobic. Among the many benefits of a plant based diet is to optimize the cellular pH.

What to Do?

- Proper diet (plant based, proper fats for conductivity through cell membranes)
- avoidance of toxins (especially too much alcohol)
- oxygenation of the cells, with proper deep breathing the oxygen and carbon dioxide ratio help in pH

Summary

This chapter is intended to be a primer and a wakeup call to the patient and physician. This chapter could have been thousands of pages long. By changing the underlying cause of your cancer, your doctor's best therapies are more likely to yield dividends on your road to recovery.

For more information about changing the underlying causes of disease go to GettingHealthier.com

PATIENT PROFILE

RM was a 20 year old white male with cancer of the mouth. His wisdom teeth had erupted sideways and continually chewed on the inside of his cheek, which is exactly where he developed cancer. His cancer was caused by chronic inflammation. His wisdom teeth were removed. He received a few doses of radiation to the region. His cancer was cured and never returned. Normally, head and neck cancers are considered "poor prognostic" cancers. For most cancer patients no one addresses the issue of "why did you get the cancer?". Let's change the etiology.

ENDNOTES

[1] https://www.ncbi.nlm.nih.gov/pubmed/8709360/
[2] https://www.ncbi.nlm.nih.gov/pubmed/18373174
[3] https://www.ncbi.nlm.nih.gov/pubmed/8237062
[4] https://www.sciencedirect.com/science/article/abs/pii/S0008621508004102
[5] https://www.ifm.org/find-a-practitioner/
[6] https://www.naturopathic.org/AF_MemberDirectory.asp?version=2
[7] http://health.lifeextension.com/InnovativeDoctors/
[8] https://jnnp.bmj.com/content/43/2/127.short
[9] https://onlinelibrary.wiley.com/doi/full/10.1111/j.1582-4934.2009.00994.x
[10] https://nutritionandmetabolism.biomedcentral.com/articles/10.1186/1743-7075-9-72
[11] https://onlinelibrary.wiley.com/doi/abs/10.1002/1097-0142(19810415)47:8%3C2026::AID-CNCR2820470821%3E3.0.CO;2-G
[12] https://link.springer.com/article/10.1007/s11523-012-0233-x
[13] https://www.psychologytoday.com/us/blog/feeling-it/201304/breathing-the-little-known-secret-peace-mind
[14] https://www.healthline.com/health/diaphragmatic-breathing

[15] https://www.cordem.org/globalassets/files/academic-assembly/2017-aa/handouts/day-three/biofeedback-exercises-for-stress-2---fernances-j.pdf

[16] https://www.ncbi.nlm.nih.gov/pmc/articles/PMC6284174/

[17] https://www.liebertpub.com/doi/abs/10.1089/thy.2005.15.1253

[18] https://link.springer.com/article/10.1007/s11892-012-0356-6

[19] http://citeseerx.ist.psu.edu/viewdoc/download?doi=10.1.1.553.1552&rep=rep1&type=pdf

[20] https://content.iospress.com/articles/biofactors/bio308

[21] https://europepmc.org/abstract/med/16498360

[22] https://onlinelibrary.wiley.com/doi/abs/10.1002/jcb.10653

[23] https://academic.oup.com/jnci/article/92/4/328/2624742

KEY 12
RATIONAL CANCER TREATMENT

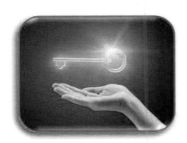

Chapter 12
Rational Cancer Treatment

"New beginnings are often disguised as painful endings."
Tao Te Ching (literally: Book of the Way and Its Virtue), circa 500 BC

FROM NATURE'S PHARMACY: Tomatoes

      The humble tomato is one of nature's more nutrient packed and cheap fruits. Tomatoes were first cultivated in Central and South America, then brought back to Europe by Spanish explorers around 1595. Europeans were leery of the tomato at first because it is a member of the nightshade plants. The leaves and unripe fruit can be toxic. The acid from the tomatoes would tint their pewter dishes. Eventually people lost their fear of tomatoes and embraced this delicious, beautiful and nutritious fruit. In 1897 soup mogul Joseph Campbell introduced tomato soup, much to the delight of his followers. Due to the high acid content of tomatoes, canning is relatively easy and safe. Given the right conditions of soil, water, sunshine, and heat; tomato plants can be prolific producers of fruit. Every year in the last week of August, which is when tomatoes are so abundant, Valencia, Spain hosts the La Tomatina festival of throwing the excess and overripe tomatoes in the world's grandest food fight. Many areas around the world have duplicated this event.

Meanwhile, tomatoes are a rich source of vitamin C, lycopene, fiber, potassium, vitamin K, naringenin, and other phytochemicals. Tomatoes are so cheap, nutritious and well-tolerated by most people that scientists who are researching the effects of antioxidants on health and disease usually use tomato paste. Tomatoes help to support the immune 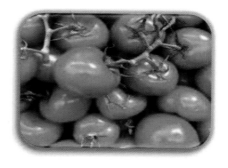 system, reduce inflammation, and reduce free radical damage in the body. 1 Tomatoes help to improve circulation and reduce the risk for stroke. 2 Tomato consumption lowers the risk for many cancers. 3 Lycopene is best absorbed when some fat is eaten at the same meal, which may be why the Mediterranean diet adds olive oil to the tomato salad. Some people react poorly to tomatoes, but that is no reason for the vast majority of the population to avoid these tasty and nourishing delights.

Changing the underlying conditions that brought on the cancer (naturopathic) and attacking the cancer with therapies that kill cancer, but do not harm the host (cytotoxic), can be an incredibly effective combination.

Chemotherapy, radiation, and surgery may be appropriate in certain cancers and for certain people. But make sure that the physician understands the concept of "restrained" medical therapies against cancer. I have worked with cancer patients who were devastated by unrestrained chemo, radiation, or surgery.

Impact of pharmacological ascorbate on tumor growth

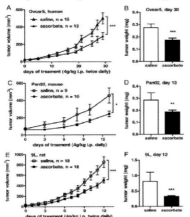

...parenteral (IV) ascorbate as the only treatment significantly decreased both tumor growth and weight by 41-53%...

metastases were absent in ascorbate treated animals...

These data suggest that ascorbate as a prodrug may have benefits in cancers with poor prognosis and limited therapeutic options.

Chen Q. et.al. PNAS 2008;105:11105-11109

@2008 by The National Academy of Sciences of the USA

PNAS

COMPREHENSIVE CANCER TREATMENT INCLUDES:

1 ↓

change underlying cause(s) of disease
NUTRITION
DETOXIFICATION
DYSBIOSIS
HORMONE BAL.
HYPERGLYCEMIA
INFECTIONS
STRESS
EXERCISE
ENERGY PATHWAYS
ETC.

2 ↓

restrained tumor debulking
CHEMO?
RADIATION
SURGERY
BURZYNSKI
HYPERTHERM
PHOTO-CYTO
HERBALS
APHERESIS
LYMPH.INFUS.

3 ↓

symptom management
PAIN**
NAUSEA
ANOREXIA
ANEMIA
LEUKOPENIA
DEPRESSION
CACHEXIA
HAIR LOSS

If you threw a hand grenade into your garage to get rid of the mice, then you may have accomplished the goal of killing the mice, but you don't have a garage anymore. Similarly, too many cancer patients are exposed to "maximum sub-lethal" therapies, which may provide an initial "response" or tumor shrinkage, but in the end may reduce the quality and quantity of life for the cancer patient by suppressing immune functions, damaging the heart and kidneys, and creating a tumor that is "drug resistant", or virtually bullet-proof.

Don't Take Your Vitamin C Unless...

A couple of hundred thousand years ago, humans lost the ability to convert blood sugar (glucose) into vitamin C (ascorbic acid). Some scientists have called this evolutionary shift a figurative "fall from the Garden of Eden". All but a few creatures on earth produce their own vitamin C in massive quantities, with higher internal production when the creature gets sick. For instance, a 150-pound goat makes about 10,000 milligrams daily of vitamin C. Meanwhile, the Recommended Dietary Allowance for a 156-pound reference human is 60 milligrams per day.

Vitamin C is one of the more utilitarian nutrients in the human body, by assisting in the construction of connective tissue (the glue that keeps the body together), regulating the levels of fats in the blood, assisting in iron absorption, aiding in the synthesis of various brain chemicals for thought, and protecting against the damaging effects of free radicals. In a study done at the University of California at Los Angeles, men who took supplements of 300 mg daily of vitamin C (5 times the RDA) lived an average of 6 years longer than men who did not take supplements of vitamin C. Mark Levine, MD, researcher with the National Institutes of Health, finds evidence that 250 mg per day might be a more rational and healthy RDA for vitamin C.

Meanwhile, oncologists worry about the possibility that vitamin C might inhibit the free radical activity of chemotherapy and radiation in destroying cancer cells. While it might seem logical that an antioxidant (like vitamin C) might reduce the effectiveness of a pro-oxidant (like chemo and radiation), the opposite has been found in animal and human studies: antioxidants protect the healthy tissue of the patient while allowing the cancer tissue to become more vulnerable to the damaging effects of chemo and radiation.

Now let me weave all of this seemingly confusing data together to help make sense for the cancer patient. Any antioxidant can become a pro-oxidant in a given chemical soup. That is why Nature always gives us droves of different antioxidants to play "hot potato" with unpaired electrons until their destructive energy is dissipated. No food has just one antioxidant. No human cell wants just one antioxidant. Antioxidants can become pro-oxidants when in isolation, which is exactly what happens to cancer cells when they selectively absorb only vitamin C, hoping to get some fuel for growth. What really happens is the vitamin C quickly becomes a pro- oxidant, targeting its destruction exclusively for the cancer cells. Dozens of very well trained physicians have been giving high doses of intravenous vitamin C (10 to 100 grams daily) to thousands of cancer patients for decades with no side effects, and usually improved outcome.[4] Intravenous vitamin C seems to have selective anti-cancer activity, according to an article in the *Annals of Internal Medicine* (Apr.6, 2004, p.533), authored by several doctors including researchers at the National Institutes of Health. IV vitamin C supports cancer patients in many well documented pathways.[5] Dr. Hugh Riordan reported improved outcome in poor prognostic cancer patients who have been put in remission through use of high dose IV vitamin C.

Vitamin C supplements can be helpful in slowing cancer, while making medical therapy more of a selective toxin against the cancer and protecting healthy host tissue. Vitamin C protects against heart disease, lengthens life span, and more...when taken in conjunction with a wide assortment of other antioxidants along with a good diet.

A number of bright researchers have taken a tiny bit of knowledge out of context (vitamin C thickens artery walls, is selectively absorbed by tumors, can become a pro-oxidant), then ASSUMED a sequence of unproven conclusions, without consulting the "prior art" in this field. Don't take your vitamin C supplements--unless you want to live longer.

Hyperthermia

When a human gets sick, mother nature triggers a fever. A fever is an extraordinary therapy to help us get well. Fevers raise the body temperature which has several major benefits, including "cooking" the pathogen above normal body temperature and reducing the viscosity of the lymphatic fluid for a more efficient flow of immune cells throughout the body.

This same fever, or <u>hyperthermia, has been used successfully</u> in many cancer patients.[6] In general, normal body temperature is 98.6 F (37 C). Hyperthermia raises body temperature to selectively kill the cancer cells. Hyperthermia can be used in combination with other medical therapies. At one time, cancer patients would be placed in a sophisticated hot tub for hyperthermia. <u>New technology uses microwaves</u> and ultrasound to generate heat.

Others

Hyperbaric oxygen, as discussed in the section on "changing the underlying conditions" can be very effective at <u>reducing tumor burden</u>.[7]

<u>High dose curcumin</u>, either orally or intravenously, can be useful against cancer.[8]

Insulin Potentiated Targeted Low Dose (IPTLD) therapy has been used with some success against cancer. There is an <u>international organization</u> of physicians who oversee this very promising therapy.[9]

<u>Ozone therapy</u> in combination with chemo and radiation has been used with some success against cancer.[10]

<u>Autohemotherapy</u> involves withdrawing some of the patient's blood, then injecting that blood, possibly after some treatment, into the patient. Autohemotherapy is an <u>exceptional treatment for shingles</u>, an infection that causes serious pain and complications in many people over age 50.[11]

<u>Pulsed electromagnetic field therapy</u> (PEMF) has been used successfully in cancer treatment.[12]

Key 12:
Selective tumor debulking
Kill the cancer, not the patient

IV vitamin C
Hyperthermia
Hyperbaric oxygen
High dose curcumin, IV or oral
IPTLD
Autohemotherapy
Ozone
PEMF

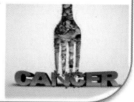

For more information about rational cancer treatment options go to GettingHealthier.com

---

PATIENT PROFILE: A LIFE WELL LIVED

"Cancer is the best thing that ever happened to me." V.G. was at the podium speaking to a hundred people at a Celebrate Life Reunion of cancer victors. V.G. had come to our hospital with stage 4 breast cancer, in great pain, and expecting imminent death. She went through our medical program while following the principles in BEATING CANCER WITH NUTRITION. V.G. had dramatic shrinkage of her tumors and went on to write THERE'S NO PLACE LIKE HOPE, which provided inspiration to thousands of her readers. V.G. lived another 14 years beyond her death sentence with relatively good quality of life. V.G. found her values and attitudes dramatically changed by her experience with cancer. In Oriental language "crisis" is written with two characters: one is "danger" and the other is "opportunity". Cancer is a life-threatening disease that presents to you the opportunity of turning your life into a masterpiece...just like V.G.

ENDNOTES

[1] https://www.ncbi.nlm.nih.gov/pubmed/16569044

[2] https://www.ncbi.nlm.nih.gov/pubmed/22969932

[3] https://www.ncbi.nlm.nih.gov/pubmed/10050865

[4] https://www.ncbi.nlm.nih.gov/pubmed/15068981

[5] https://www.ncbi.nlm.nih.gov/pmc/articles/PMC5927785/

[6] https://www.sciencedirect.com/science/article/abs/pii/S1470204502008185

[7] https://link.springer.com/article/10.1007/s11523-012-0233-x

[8] https://clincancerres.aacrjournals.org/content/14/14/4491.short

[9] http://iptldacademy.org/

[10] https://www.ncbi.nlm.nih.gov/pmc/articles/PMC6151231/

[11] https://www.liebertpub.com/doi/abs/10.1089/acm.1997.3.155

[12] https://www.ncbi.nlm.nih.gov/pmc/articles/PMC5119968/